This wonderful tool finally gives us the opportunity to really understand carbohydrate counting and its application to diabetes management. It is clear, concise, and easy to understand and apply. It will be very beneficial to health care professionals and people with diabetes.

Ginger Kanzer-Lewis
President, American Association of Diabetes Educators

This is an excellent resource for both health professionals and people with diabetes who want to know how to have maximum flexibility in meal planning while achieving excellent blood glucose control.

Virginia Valentine, MS, RN, CDE

A wonderfully practical, step-by-step guide to using carbohydrate counting.

Anne Daly, MS, RD, LD, CDE

This book got me off the roller coaster and put me back in the driver's seat! It helps you understand the big picture— the relationship between nutrition, diabetes medications, and exercise—so that you can balance your diabetes confidently.

J. Scott Rainey, person with diabetes

An excellent how-to guide for anyone needing flexible food choices...

Midwest Book Review

Complete Guide
to Carb
Counting

Hope S. Warshaw, MMSc, RD, CDE
Karmeen Kulkarni, MS, RD, CDE

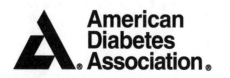

American
Diabetes
Association®

Director, Book Publishing, John Fedor; *Editor*, Sherrye L. Landrum; *Production Manager*, Peggy M. Rote; *Composition*, Circle Graphics, Inc.; *Cover Design*, VC Graphics Design Studio, Inc.; *Printer*, Transcontinental Printing

Printed in Canada
3 5 7 9 10 8 6 4 2

The suggestions and information contained in this publication are generally consistent with the *Clinical Practice Recommendations* and other policies of the American Diabetes Association, but they do not represent the policy or position of the Association or any of its boards or committees. Reasonable steps have been taken to ensure the accuracy of the information presented. However, the American Diabetes Association cannot ensure the safety or efficacy of any product or service described in this publication. Individuals are advised to consult a physician or other appropriate health care professional before undertaking any diet or exercise program or taking any medication referred to in this publication. Professionals must use and apply their own professional judgment, experience, and training and should not rely solely on the information contained in this publication before prescribing any diet, exercise, or medication. The American Diabetes Association—its officers, directors, employees, volunteers, and members—assumes no responsibility or liability for personal or other injury, loss, or damage that may result from the suggestions or information in this publication.

♾ The paper in this publication meets the requirements of the ANSI Standard Z39.48-1992 (permanence of paper).

ADA titles may be purchased for business or promotional use or for special sales. For information, please write to Lee Romano Sequeira, Special Sales & Promotions, at the address below.

American Diabetes Association
1701 North Beauregard Street
Alexandria, Virginia 22311

Library of Congress Cataloging-in-Publication Data
Warshaw, Hope S., 1954-
    Complete guide to carb counting / Hope S. Warshaw, Karmeen Kulkarni.
    p. cm.
    Includes index.
    ISBN 1-58040-046-9 (pbk. : alk. paper)
    1. Diabetes–Diet therapy. 2. Food–Carbohydrate content. I. Kulkarni,
Karmeen, 1953- II. Title.
    RC662 .W313 2001
    616.4'620654–dc21
                                                        2001022562

*This book is dedicated to all people with diabetes.
We hope it provides you with the
knowledge and skills to
make carb counting a central part of
your diabetes care and
helps you to achieve the diabetes control and
quality of life that you desire.*

Contents

Foreword

Choosing what to eat when you have diabetes can be a challenge. You have to carefully balance food, medication, and activity to get the best glucose control possible. Carbohydrate counting is one of several meal planning approaches that you can use to help you know what and how much you should eat.

The Diabetes Control and Complications Trial (DCCT) results that were announced in 1993 proved that good diabetes control significantly reduces development of long-term complications. Participants in the DCCT used carb counting. Since then, more and more people with diabetes have turned to carbohydrate counting to help them make food choices, both because of their desire for tight blood glucose control and for flexibility in food choices and lifestyle. But to learn to use carbohydrate counting means you learn to think and speak in "carbohydrate language." The more you practice, the more fluent you become, and eventually you become skilled in carbohydrate counting.

This book is a practical and comprehensive step-by-step guide to using carbohydrate counting. The authors begin with the basics—why count carbohydrate and what foods contain carbohydrate. Then they explain how to plan meals and snacks using carbohydrate counting and emphasize how very important portion sizes are. They give you tools, tips, and tricks to help you get the correct size portions wherever you are. They discuss the effect of protein and fat on blood glucose control, how to use food labels, and how to eat out in restaurants, especially in this super-sized world.

You'll need to keep records to learn and practice carbohydrate counting, because your records provide feedback about how your blood glucose is affected by food, medication, and activity. Learning to see patterns in the records and to make adjustments to solve problems is all part of carb counting. With practice, you can develop advanced skills and determine the amount of insulin you need to cover the food you eat, usually using a ratio of insulin to grams of carbohydrate eaten.

This book is a great help to people who want to learn about carbohydrate counting for the first time or to fine-tune their carb counting skills to get the best blood glucose control possible. You will gain the confidence to manage your diabetes in new ways, along with great potential for improving your overall health today and tomorrow.

Anne Daly, MS, RD, LD, CDE
President, Health Care & Education
American Diabetes Association

Acknowledgments

Thanks to several colleagues who provided valuable critiques: Sandy Gillespie, MMSc, RD, CDE, and David Shade, MD. Thanks to Anne Daly, MS, RD, CDE, for reviewing the manuscript and writing the Foreword. Thanks to Virginia Valentine, MS, RD, CDE; Ginger Kanzer Lewis, MS, RD, CDE; and Nicole Johnson for their review and quotes. The authors also thank J. Scott Rainey, a patient with type 1 diabetes, for his thorough review and thoughtful comments.

Thanks to the staff at ADA—Sherrye, Peggy, Keith, and Lee—who helped to edit and prepare the manuscript for printing and developed marketing and publicity to ensure the success of this book.

1

Why Count Carbs?

Would you like to know when your blood sugar is going to rise—and more than that, about how high it's going to go? Would you like to know what your blood sugars will do tomorrow and the next day and the next? Well, counting carbohydrates can provide you with answers and help you gain better control of your blood sugar levels than ever before.

Food contains carbohydrate, protein, fat, vitamins, minerals, and water. So, why do we only count carbohydrate? Because it is the carbohydrate in foods that raises your blood sugar the most. Simply put, you count the carbohydrate in the cereal, banana, and milk that you ate for breakfast, and check how high your blood glucose is 1–2 hours later. The next morning you eat the same amount of cereal, banana, and milk. And lo and behold, when you check 1–2 hours later, your blood sugar is at the same level it was yesterday! The first two mornings you don't do any exercise, but you do take your diabetes medication. The third morning after you eat your cereal and banana breakfast, you take a walk. Surprise! Your blood sugar level 1–2 hours later is not the same—it's lower than on the other days. You can see that carbs raise your blood sugar but exercise and diabetes medications lower it.

You can eat cereal and banana for breakfast from now on and find your blood sugar levels falling into a predictable pattern. But what if you get tired of eating cereal and banana? Tomorrow you may want a waffle, orange juice, and a piece of bacon. The next day you might eat a breakfast of scrambled egg, hash-brown potatoes, and toast. First count the grams of carbohydrate in the cereal, banana, and milk. If the other breakfasts contain the same number of grams of carbohydrate as the cereal breakfast, your blood sugar is going up the same amount as it did with the cereal. It's the carbohydrates that count.

Getting to Choose

Some people with diabetes are afraid to change their meal plans. They won't go out to eat, and eat the same foods over and over. But if you count the carbs in them, you can add new foods to breakfast, lunch, and dinner menus without having to risk unexpected high blood sugar levels. Carb counting is a way to focus your diabetes management and get a new variety of foods on your plate each day. Being consistent is the key. If you eat about the same amount of carbohydrate at each meal and snack each day, your blood sugars are more likely to fall into a steady pattern, which means better diabetes control for you. You CAN take some of the mystery out of what is going to happen to your blood sugar.

If you have a meal plan, it may suggest 45 grams (g) of carbohydrate at breakfast, 60 g of carb at lunch, 15 g in a mid-afternoon snack, and 70 g at dinner, with perhaps another 15 g for your bedtime snack, if you're having frequent low blood sugar levels in the middle of the night. Uh oh, your meal plan isn't written in grams of carbohydrate? It uses servings from food groups on the Food Guide Pyramid or the Exchange Lists? That's okay, you can quickly learn that a serving of bread has 15 g of carbohydrate and a serving of vegetables has 5 g of carbohydrate and a serving of meat has 0 g of carbohydrate. There are many resources to help you find out how much carbohydrate is in the food you're eating, but before you can count carbs, you need to know what foods contain them.

Which foods contain carbohydrate?

Bet your answer is starches, such as potatoes and corn. Then you add bread, cereal, rice, crackers, and pasta. Oh, and don't forget the starchy vegetables—peas, beans, and lentils. If you're like most people, that's where you stop, so it may surprise you to learn that a number of other foods contain carbohydrate, too:

- fruit and fruit juice
- vegetables
- milk and yogurt
- cheese
- sugary foods, such as candy and regular soda
- sweets, such as cakes, cookies, and pies

How much carbohydrate is in it?

Table 1-1 lists average amounts of carbohydrate in some common foods so you can begin to practice carb counting. Check to see how many carbs are in a typical commercial slice of bread—15 grams of carbohydrate. Appendix 1 lists the amount of carbohydrate in many other foods. Appendix 2 gives you a list of books and other resources where you can find the amount of carbohydrate in many more foods— from apples to zabaglione. This is important information for you—especially if you eat foods that don't have food labels, such as fresh fruit and vegetables or fast foods.

Please note that meats and fats don't contain carbohydrate, so you don't count them. This doesn't mean that you ignore protein and fat (see chapter 6). Vegetables

TABLE 1-1 Nutrients				
Food group	Serving*	Carbohydrate (g)	Protein (g)	Fat (g)
Bread	1 slice	15	3	0
Cereal, dry	1 oz	15	3	†
Cereal, cooked	1/2 cup	15	3	†
Pasta, cooked	1/2 cup	15	3	†
Starchy vegetable	1/3 to 1/2 cup	15	3	0
Fruit, fresh	1 medium piece	15	0	0
Fruit, canned, no sugar added	1/2 cup	15	0	0
Vegetables	1/2 cup cooked	5	0	0
Vegetable	1 cup raw	5	0	0
Milk, fat free	1 cup	12	8	0
Yogurt, plain, nonfat	3/4 cup	12	8	0
Sugary foods	1 serving	Varies	Varies	Varies
Sweets	1 serving	Varies	Varies	Varies
Meats	3 oz cooked	0	21	Varies
Fats— margarine, mayonnaise, oil	1 tsp	0	0	5

* Servings are from *Exchange Lists for Meal Planning* published by ADA and The American Dietetic Association, 1995.
† Depends on the product.

contain a little carbohydrate (and a lot of vitamins and minerals), so you can eat big servings of them.

Size Does Count

You might want to look at carb counting as a personal science experiment. You'll find there's never been a better subject to study than yourself. To get information that you can use, you must measure the ingredients (foods) carefully. That's why we begin by focusing on the size of your servings. This seems so simple, but even dietitians have to take this basic step. Take out the bowl and plate and cup that you usually use. Now get a measuring cup and see how much cereal your bowl actually holds. Are you eating a 1/2 cup serving of oatmeal or a 2-cup serving of oatmeal every day? Looking at the chart, you see that the 1/2 cup serving has 15 g of carbohydrate in it. The 2 cups that you actually eat have 4 times as much carbohydrate or 60 grams of carbohydrate. This makes a big difference to your blood sugar level when that carbohydrate is digested!

Many people with diabetes don't understand portion sizes, which can lead to poor blood glucose control. The most powerful step that you can take to balance your blood sugar (and your weight) is to measure your serving sizes—and to eat that serving. (How many servings are you eating?) This will work even with the foods that aren't on your meal plan. For example, if you're eating a 2-cup bowl of ice cream every night, it will be an improvement for your health if you measure out 1 cup and eat it. (In case you were wondering, you can substitute the carbs in the ice cream for some other carbohydrate in your meal plan, such as potatoes or bread at dinner. More about this later.)

How does carb counting help with blood sugar control?

You can count the carbs in every food you eat for the rest of your life, but unless you make some notes about how they affect your blood sugar level, you won't have the information you need. What's on your fork? Write it down. What's your blood glucose? Write it down. The first few weeks of carb counting are the science experiment—perhaps the most important one you'll ever do. With carb counting, curiosity definitely pays off.

Check Appendix 3 for a record-keeping form that you might use. For a few weeks you write down the grams of carbohydrate in each food you eat, check your blood sugar level 1–2 hours after you eat, and record that number, too. (Be sure to list any carbohydrate you eat to bring up blood sugar that is too low.) List the dose of diabetes medication that you usually take or the extra that you had to take to bring your blood sugar level back to normal. Write any physical activity into the record (which lowers blood sugar) and any stressful situations that pop up, such as getting the flu or getting into a heated argument (which usually raise blood sugar). We know that all these factors influence blood sugar levels, but this research will tell you how they affect your own blood sugar levels. The more you find out about how other factors affect your blood sugar, the more you benefit from this experiment.

After keeping your records for several weeks, you can begin to look for patterns in your blood sugar numbers— your own patterns. Each person has a blood glucose (glycemic) response to different foods. You need to know what yours is. For example, your records may tell you that a slice of pizza raises your blood sugar by so many points, and a certain amount of medication and/or exercise brings it back to normal.

What's so important about controlling blood glucose levels?

When you keep your blood glucose levels nearer normal, you feel better today and help prevent or delay long-term complications of diabetes.

Table 1-2 gives you the blood glucose levels that the American Diabetes Association (ADA) recommends for people with diabetes. Discuss your target levels with your health care provider because yours may be different from the ones in the table. For example, a pregnant woman may have lower target levels and an older person at risk for having a stroke may have higher target levels than those in Table 1-2. In general, if you keep your blood glucose levels and hemoglobin A_{1c} (the 3-month average of your blood

TABLE 1-2 Target Ranges for Blood Glucose and Hemoglobin A$_{1c}$ Levels

	Goal
Whole blood values	
Average before meal glucose (mg/dl)	80–120
Average bedtime glucose (mg/dl)	100–140
2 hours after meals (mg/dl)	160–180*
Plasma values	
Average before meal glucose (mg/dl)	90–130
Average bedtime glucose (mg/dl)	110–130
2 hours after meals (mg/dl)	170–190*
Hemoglobin A$_{1c}$ (HbA$_{1c}$) (%)	<7

* No ADA recommendation exists for after-meal blood glucose levels. These recommendations come from consensus among diabetes care providers. You check 2 hours after the beginning of the meal.

glucose levels) in your target ranges, you have the best chance at feeling good today and staying healthy for the rest of your life.

Check to see whether your meter measures the amount of blood glucose in whole blood or in plasma. Plasma is more concentrated, so those levels are higher than the whole blood values.

Basic Facts about Carbohydrate

All the carbohydrate you eat is broken down into glucose (sugar) about 2 hours from the time you start eating. Carbohydrates are the body's main and preferred energy source. There are two categories of carbohydrates: complex and simple. Complex carbs have many sugar units, or saccharides, hooked together. Some of the complex carbohydrates you eat are grains, pasta, and potatoes. Simple carbohydrates have just two sugar units, or saccharides, hooked together. You eat simple carbohydrates in fruit, fruit juice, and regular soda.

Once you eat any type of carb, it is broken down into one-unit sugars (glucose) that goes into your bloodstream. With the help of the hormone insulin, the cells of your body can use the glucose in your blood for energy. At that point, your body doesn't know whether the sugar came from mashed potatoes or a piece of apple pie. All carbohydrates become glucose—the body's favorite source of energy.

Should you eat carbs?

Yes. Once you realize the impact that carbohydrates have on your blood glucose, you might jump to the conclusion that it's best to steer clear of them. Please don't skimp on carbohydrates, because foods with carbohydrate are among the healthiest foods you can eat. Unless you add fat to them, carbs have very little fat—consider a bowl of pasta, a banana, a glass of fat-free milk, vegetables, fruit, or whole grains. These foods also contain essential vitamins and minerals you don't get in other foods, and your body needs them to be healthy. Carbs also contain fiber that is very important in keeping your body healthy. And your body prefers to use carbohydrate as its source of energy!

What about sugars?

Some sugars occur naturally in foods, such as the fructose in fruit and the lactose in milk. Other sugars—such as sucrose (table sugar) or corn syrup—are added to foods when they are processed. The most important thing about sugars is that they are carbohydrate and will raise your blood glucose. When you eat any of the following, remember to count the carbohydrates in them:

- Sweeteners you find in your pantry—granulated sugar, brown sugar, honey, maple syrup—and the sweeteners used in commercial food products that you see on the food label—high-fructose corn syrup, corn sweeteners, and dextrose.

- Sugary foods such as regular soda, candy, jelly, and sweetened fruit drinks.

- Sweets such as cake, cookies, pie, candy, and desserts. Sweets usually also contain fat, and lots of calories, but for carb counting, we focus on the carbohydrates that will raise your blood glucose level.

When can you eat sugary foods and sweets?

When you substitute them into your meal plan for other carbohydrates or adjust your diabetes medications to account for the extra carbohydrate. This may be a difficult concept for people with diabetes to accept (or for your friends and family). Are we saying that you can eat all the desserts you want? No, we are not suggesting that you have sweets every day. We are suggesting that you can learn how to work sweets into your eating plan.

Throughout the 20th century, the most widely held belief about what to eat when you have diabetes was to "avoid sugar." The carbs to eat were bread, potatoes, and rice. However, in the past 20 years, we've found very little scientific evidence to support this idea. In fact, fruits and milk have been shown to have a lower effect on blood glucose than bread, potatoes, or beans. Table sugar has about the same effect on blood glucose that bread, rice, and potatoes do. So, what's important for controlling your blood glucose level is the **total amount of carbohydrate in the meal—not the type of food you eat.**

So what's wrong with sugary foods and sweets? They have lots of calories but very few vitamins and minerals— empty calories. In our country, most people eat too much sugar and too many calories. All Americans are being encouraged to eat more nutritious foods such as vegetables because they have lots of vitamins and minerals and few

- Choose a few favorite desserts and decide how often to eat them.

- Satisfy your sweet tooth with a bite or two of your favorite sweet.

- If you have a difficult time limiting portions or how often you eat sweets, it is best not to bring large portions of sweets into the house. You might only order dessert at restaurants or just purchase a small quantity at a time.

- Split a dessert with a dining companion in a restaurant. Ask for several forks or spoons.

- Take advantage of smaller portions—kiddie, small, or regular—at ice cream shops or in the supermarket.

- Check your blood glucose from time to time 1–2 hours after you eat a sweet to see how high it makes your blood glucose rise.

calories. In fact, the 2000 Dietary Guideline about sugars from the United States Department of Agriculture advises everyone to choose foods and beverages so we get smaller amounts of sugars.

If you simply are not a sweets eater, then continue to steer clear of them. If, on the other hand, you can't live without them, go ahead and enjoy them once in a while. Here are the American Diabetes Association's general guidelines for eating sugary foods and sweets:

- Substitute sugary foods or sweets for other carbohydrates in your meal plan.

- If you chose to eat a sweet, then lighten up on other carbohydrates in the meal—for example, have smaller or fewer servings of bread, potato, or fruit.

EASY WAYS TO REDUCE SUGARS

- Trade regular soda for diet soda, or even better, water.

- When you order or buy iced tea, make sure it is unsweetened or sweetened with a low-calorie sweetener.

- When you buy fruit drinks or flavored seltzers, read the Nutrition Facts. Make sure the calories, carbohydrate, and sugars are near zero. You can substitute fruit drink for fruit juice, but it's better to drink water and eat pieces of fruit.

- Trade canned fruit packed in heavy syrup for fruit packed in its own juice or light syrup.

- Use low-calorie sweetener instead of sugar.

- Use low- or no-sugar jelly or jam instead of regular.

▪ Burn the extra calories from sweets with more exercise. (How long do you need to walk to balance the effects of that doughnut?)

Think about these points to help you decide how often to eat sugary foods and sweets.

▪ Limit sugary and sweet foods until you get your blood glucose and hemoglobin A_{1c} under control.

▪ If one of your goals is to lose some weight, then you'll need to keep sweets to a once-in-a-while frequency. Too many sweets equals too many calories.

▪ If your total cholesterol, LDL, HDL, and triglycerides are out of control, we recommend that you keep sweets to a minimum because sweets contain fats. Get your blood fats close to normal before you add more sweets to your meal plan (see chapter 6).

■ What triggers you to want to eat sweets? Think about how much you enjoy sweets and how often you want to eat them. Can you use this information to create realistic diabetes, nutrition, and health goals?

Fiber and Blood Glucose

The fiber in foods, called dietary fiber, is another source of carbohydrate. The main sources of fiber are foods that contain most of their calories from carbohydrate—whole grains, breads, cereals, beans and peas, and fruits and vegetables. Fiber can affect how quickly your food is digested and can have an effect on your blood glucose level as well. There are two types of dietary fiber—insoluble and soluble.

Insoluble fibers. Insoluble fibers give form to foods. Foods that contain insoluble fiber are whole grain cereals and breads. Insoluble fibers grab onto liquid as they travel down the gastrointestinal tract. That's good because the combination of fiber and liquid pushes food through the gastrointestinal tract more quickly. If you eat a good supply of insoluble fiber to promote a bulkier and softer bowel movement, you also reap other health benefits—preventing hemorrhoids, diverticulosis, and colon and rectal cancer.

Soluble fiber. Soluble fibers dissolve during digestion but remain gummy and thick. Food sources of soluble fiber are beans, peas, and some grains, such as oats and barley. The benefits of soluble fiber are different from insoluble fibers. The soluble fibers can prevent the body from absorbing certain nutrients in foods. Two important ones are cholesterol and glucose. It is thought that eating a lot of soluble fiber can, by binding onto cholesterol during digestion, lower blood cholesterol a small amount. It is also thought that eating a lot of soluble fiber can lower the rise of blood glucose by slowing down the absorption of glucose. But you have to eat a very large amount of soluble fiber to get that reaction.

The ADA says it is doubtful that people can eat enough soluble fiber daily to have any great effect on lowering blood glucose or improving lipid levels. But ADA does recognize the health benefits of eating fiber and recommends that you eat plenty—20–35 grams from both soluble and insoluble fibers from a wide variety of food sources daily. (Most Americans only eat about 14 grams of fiber a day.) You can have some fun finding ways to get more fiber in your meals.

Q: What is the Glycemic Index and does it apply to carb counting?

R: The Glycemic Index of foods is a list of foods and how they affect blood glucose levels. It was developed in the early 1980s by researchers who studied how quickly or slowly various carbohydrate-containing foods raised blood glucose—bread, corn, pasta, beans, fruit, and others. The glycemic index research helped to show that not all carbohydrates raise blood glucose levels the same amount. They showed, for instance, that potatoes raised blood glucose more quickly than fruit and that legumes raised blood glucose quite slowly.

This was valuable research, but this method is not so useful to you at home because it looks at only one food at a time. This is not how people really eat. Most people eat several foods in a meal, and some are high in carbohydrate while others are high in protein or fat. In addition, a number of other factors affect how quickly foods raise blood glucose, such as

- how much blood glucose–lowering medication you take
- the time of your last dose of diabetes medication and the time you eat
- the fiber content of the foods you eat
- the ripeness of the fruit or vegetable you eat
- whether the food is cooked or raw

- how quickly or slowly you eat

- level of blood glucose (rises faster when blood glucose is low)

Although some health care practitioners, particularly in Australia, and people with diabetes use the Glycemic Index for meal planning, the ADA has not endorsed it. That's because of the many other factors that affect the rise in blood glucose levels. Besides, if people with diabetes only eat foods that cause a low glycemic rise, they limit their food choices and risk losing variety in their meals. Eating a variety of foods is the number one guideline for people who want to be healthy. No doubt it is healthy to eat many of the low glycemic foods, such as whole grains and legumes, but you also need the foods with a high glycemic index, such as pasta and fruit.

That said, in a sense, you will develop your own glycemic index as you progress with carb counting. You'll be keeping records of the foods you eat, their affect on your blood glucose levels, the medication you take, the exercise you do, and the stress in your day, and the times that all this happens. You will find foods that cause your blood glucose levels to rise more than you expect. Or you might find one or more foods that raise your blood glucose very quickly. It's great to identify these foods for yourself. You may want to write them down in your personal Glycemic Index.

With this information, you can decide whether to eat a food or to eat a smaller serving. Or you might decide to take more diabetes medication to decrease the rise in your blood glucose from particular foods. However, don't be quick to jump to conclusions. Try the food several times and make sure your blood glucose isn't rising quickly or so high because the serving is too large or other foods you ate at the same time affected your blood glucose, too. See chapter 10 to learn more about using your personal experiences with foods.

Q: Doesn't it make sense for me to follow a low-carb, high-protein diet?

R: The answer is NO. What makes sense is to measure the serving sizes of your carbohydrate foods, so you're not eating too much of them. Every few years it seems that a new crop of low-carb, high-protein diets show up in best-selling books. This is because Americans want to believe that the next diet will be the magic bullet that will help them take unwanted weight off and keep it off. Beware of any diet that promises rapid weight loss, sells a product, or omits foods you know are healthy. In general, low-carb, high-protein diets are not a healthy or sensible way to eat for the rest of your life. Researchers agree that there are many health benefits from eating carbohydrates—whole grains, fruits, vegetables, and low-fat or nonfat dairy foods. Don't take them out of your diet—just measure your servings.

There is also concern that some of the low-carb diets encourage people to eat a large amount of red meats and animal fats—saturated fat. Diabetes raises your risk of having a heart attack and problems with your arteries. Eating a lot of saturated fat can increase your risk, which is why one of the strongest ADA nutrition recommendations is to keep the amount of saturated fat you eat low (about 10% of your daily calories).

Perhaps most important, none of the low-carb diets help people learn to change their eating habits enough to successfully keep weight off. It's just not so easy! The key to successful weight loss never changes: eat healthy servings of a variety of foods and get your body moving in physical activity every day.

2

What's Carb Counting?

A Bit of History

For years carbohydrate counting was the method of choice in the United Kingdom. Then in the early 1990s, carb counting got lots of attention in the Diabetes Control and Complications Trial (DCCT). This was the 10-year study of people with type 1 diabetes that showed good control of blood glucose reduces diabetes complications, such as eye, kidney, and nerve disease. Carb counting was one of the meal planning methods used in the DCCT.

Interest in carb counting also grew when the ADA used the science supporting it to make their 1994 Nutrition Recommendations. The bottom line for blood glucose control is to focus on **the total amount of carbohydrate you eat—not the source of the carbohydrate.** As far as your blood glucose level is concerned, a carbohydrate is a carbohydrate is a carbohydrate. Today many health professionals are teaching people with diabetes how to use carb counting. This method gives you flexibility in food choices and timing of your meals and improves your blood glucose control.

Basic Carb Counting

Carb counting goes from basic to advanced, and you can stop anywhere along the way. Basic carb counting is easier to follow. To put it into practice, you learn how to count the amount of carbohydrate in different foods. Then you learn how much carbohydrate you need to eat at meals and snacks. The main point of basic carb counting is to eat about the same amount of carbohydrate at the same times each day to keep your blood glucose levels in your target range.

Basic carb counting is a good meal planning approach if you have type 2 diabetes and take no diabetes medication or one or two types of diabetes pills. It is also a good starting point for people who take several shots of insulin a day, wear an insulin pump, or want to keep tight tabs on their blood glucose levels. If you take 3 or more shots of insulin per day or use a pump, you will probably want to move on to advanced carb counting to fine-tune your blood glucose control.

Meet Joe   Joe recently found out he had diabetes when he went to see his doctor about some symptoms that were bothering him. He thought he might have diabetes because several of his family members do. Joe works hard as an airplane mechanic at the local airport. Joe's blood glucose levels were in the 250 mg/dl range when he was diagnosed. His HbA$_{1c}$ was 10.5%. Joe is 56 years old and about 30 pounds overweight. He has put on about 5 pounds a year for the last 15 years. Joe also has high blood pressure, which he controls with medication. His doctor put him on a diabetes medication to help lower his blood glucose. At the same time, the doctor wrote a prescription for him to see a dietitian who specializes in working with people with diabetes. Joe made an appointment and went with his wife to see the dietitian.

The dietitian spent a lot of time talking to Joe about his eating habits and wanted to know which ones he was willing to change. Joe said that he probably needs to eat at regular times during the day and eat less food for dinner and during the evening. He thought he could give up some of his sweets as long as he was able to have a few servings each week. The dietitian thought Joe would do well with basic carbohydrate counting, but he and his wife didn't know much about nutrition. In the first session, the dietitian taught them

1. the effect of carbohydrate on blood glucose
2. what foods contain carbohydrate
3. what is a serving of carbohydrate
4. how much carbohydrate Joe should eat for breakfast, lunch, dinner, and nighttime snack

The dietitian also gave Joe some sample meals and showed him how to find the amount of total carbohydrate on the Nutrition Facts panels on foods. She suggested that he check his blood glucose two times a day at different times, including before and after meals to see the effect of carbohydrate on his blood glucose levels.

Joe's carbohydrate-based meal plan was:

Breakfast: 5 carb choices or 75 g carb

Lunch: 6 carb choices or 90 g carb

Dinner: 6 carb choices or 90 g carb

Snack: 2 carb choices or 30 g carb

Sample 1-day meal plan

Breakfast:	2 slices whole wheat toast with peanut butter	(2 carb choices/ 30 g carb)
	1 whole large banana	(2 carb choices/ 30 g carb)
	1/2 cup orange juice	(1 carb choice/ 15 g carb)
Lunch:	(Fast food restaurant) 1 hamburger	(2 carb choices/ 30 g carb)
	1 small French fries	(2 carb choices/ 30 g carb)

	1 8 oz carton fat-free milk	(1 carb choice/ 15 g carb)
	1 small peach or pear (he takes it with him)	(1 carb choice/ 15 g carb)
Dinner:	Salad 1/2 cup cooked green or yellow vegetable	
	2 cups pasta	(4 carb choices/ 60 g carb)
	1/2 cup tomato and meat sauce	(1 carb choice/ 15 g carb)
	1 dinner roll	(1 carb choice/ 15 g carb)
Snack:	1 cup fat-free milk	(1 carb choices/ 12 g carb)
	2 small cookies	(1 carb choice/ 15 g carb)

Joe scheduled another appointment in one month. He was quite pleased with himself on his return. He had lost 2 pounds and most importantly, his blood glucose levels had dropped into the mid-100s when fasting and before meals, and they were 180–200 mg/dl 2 hours after eating. But he told the dietitian that he was hungry, particularly in the evenings. In the past, this has been his munching time. They discussed whether Joe felt he needed more food or whether he was just hungry because he was used to eating then. They reworked his carb choices to give Joe more food at lunch and dinner and less at breakfast. The dietitian suggested some evening snacks that might be more satisfying.

At the dietitian's suggestion, Joe had brought in some food labels from the foods he regularly eats. They talked about how Joe could fit these foods into his carbohydrate count. The dietitian told Joe that he could burn calories and lower his blood glucose if he took a walk in the evening several nights a week. This also helps distract him from thinking too much about food. He said he was willing to take a walk three nights a week. They set up another appointment for a month later. At that time they will continue to monitor how his carbohydrate counting plan is working for Joe and his diabetes. They will also determine what else he needs to learn and what support he needs.

Basic carbohydrate counting fits Joe's needs. He finds it easy to follow, and he doesn't want to fuss with too many calculations. His blood glucose is coming into a good range using this approach and that is what is key.

Advanced Carb Counting. Advanced carb counting is more complex. You need to learn to adjust the dosage of diabetes medication(s) you take based on your blood glucose level before the meal and the amount of carbohydrate you plan to eat. You need to know the carbohydrate content of the food. You also will need to work out your "insulin-to-carbohydrate ratio" with your health care professionals. This ratio tells you how much insulin you need to take "to cover" the amount of carbohydrate you eat, so you can keep your blood glucose levels in your target range—not too high and not too low. For example, you might learn you need 1 unit of rapid-acting insulin to handle the blood glucose rise from 15 grams of carbohydrate and that 15 grams of carbohydrate usually raises your blood glucose about 50 points.

Basic and advanced carbohydrate counting are not two different meal planning approaches, but one approach that becomes more precise. The adjustments you learn to make in advanced carb counting help you manage your blood glucose levels more closely. You decide how far you want to advance. Perhaps, like Joe, you master basic carbohydrate counting and that helps you control your blood glucose levels. Then you reach a point several (or many) years later when you find that to keep your blood glucose in control you have to start taking insulin—40% of people with type 2 do move on to taking insulin as their diabetes progresses. You may have difficulty controlling your blood glucose levels on insulin, and wonder whether you can achieve better control if you learn to adjust the amount of insulin you take at each meal. Just remember that you must master the concepts of basic carbohydrate counting before you can move on to advanced carb counting.

Two Ways to Count

As you saw in Joe's meal plan, there are two ways to count carbohydrates—counting *grams* of carbohydrate or counting carbohydrate *choices*. If you learn to count grams of carbohydrate, you add up the number of grams of carbohydrate in each food you eat. It helps if you learn some shortcuts, such as the amount of carbohydrate in common foods. For example, 1/2 cup of mashed potatoes, 1 ounce of dry cereal, and 1 slice of bread all have 15 grams of carbohydrate. If you have 1 cup of mashed potatoes, you need to add 15 g and 15 g for your serving of 30 grams of carbohydrate. You can get carb counts from the Nutrition Facts panel on food labels, from carb and fat gram books, and from other resources that list the amount of carbohydrate in foods (Appendix 2). Counting the grams of carbohydrate is more precise and, therefore, more flexible. This is particularly important if you are doing advanced carb counting.

If you count carb choices, you use the exchange system food lists. One carbohydrate choice or serving has 15 grams of carbohydrate. This book uses both methods of counting but emphasizes counting the grams of carbohydrate because that is more precise. What do you do when a serving of food contains between 1 and 2 carb choices—for example, 22 grams? Having to add 1 1/2 carb choices to other fractions of carb choices is no fun. Counting actual grams of carbohydrate can be easier.

Remember the Number 15

The number 15 is a vital number when you use either method of carb counting. That's because it is the number of grams of carbohydrate in one serving (in the Exchange System) of several of the carbohydrate-containing food groups—starches, fruit, and milk and yogurt. Even though milk has only 12 g carb in a cup, we still say that one serving of milk is equal to one serving of starch or of fruit (Table 2-1).

But not all servings contain exactly 15 grams of carbohydrate. Not in the real world, at least. So, you will find that the number of grams of carbohydrate will vary from serving to serving, from food to food. To help you decide how many carbs or carb choices there are in your serving, use Table 2-2.

How much carbohydrate should you eat?

There is no set amount of carbohydrate that is right for everyone. The amount of carbohydrate you need to eat at your meals and snacks should be based on several factors:

- Your height and weight
- Your usual food habits and daily schedule
- The foods you like to eat
- The amount of physical activity you do
- Your health status and diabetes goals
- The diabetes medications you take and the times that you take them
- Your blood glucose monitoring results

TABLE 2-1 Servings of 15 Grams of Carbohydrate*			
Food group	1 serving	2 servings	3 servings
Starches	15 g	30 g	45 g
Fruit	15 g	30 g	45 g
Milk and yogurt	12 g	24 g	36 g

* Based on servings from *Exchange Lists for Meal Planning*, ADA and The American Dietetic Association, 1995.

TABLE 2-2 Carbohydrate Choices and Grams of Carbohydrate

Carbohydrate choices	Grams of carbohydrate	Grams of carbohydrate per carbohydrate choice
1/2	6–7	6–7
1	15	8–22
2	30	23–37
3	45	38–52
4	60	53–65
5	75	68–82
6	90	83–95

WHAT ARE GRAMS OF CARBOHYDRATE?

Don't confuse gram weight with carbohydrate grams.

Answer these True/False questions to check your knowledge of grams.

A gram is a unit of weight in the metric system.   **True.**

Carbohydrate is counted in grams (g).   **True.**

When you weigh something that is 1 oz, the metric conversion is 30 grams.   **True.**

You can weigh a food with carbohydrate in it and know the grams of carbohydrate.   **False.**

The number of grams of carbohydrate, protein, and fat in a food is not the same as the weight of the food itself. For example, a medium (4 oz) apple may weigh 160 grams (30 grams × 4 oz), but the amount of carbohydrate in it is about 15 grams. A medium (6 oz) potato weighs 180 grams (30 g × 6 oz), but the amount of carbohydrate in it is about 30 grams.

There are general guidelines about how to choose a level of grams of carbohydrate to eat based on whether you are male or female, small or large, and want to lose weight or not. Table 2-3 can help you design a healthy meal plan. Once you identify what is best for you, divide the servings into meals and snacks. As a starting point, most adults need 4–5 carbohydrate servings at each meal. If you take insulin, you can learn to adjust the dose to a varied amount of carbohydrate intake, but oral medications are not so easy to adjust. For people using basic carb counting, it is important to keep the amount of carbohydrate you eat at meals and snacks about the same day to day. This helps you control your blood glucose.

Consider the amount of carbohydrate suggested in Table 2-3 as a starting point. Find a dietitian who specializes in diabetes care to work with you to determine the amount of carbohydrate that best fits your needs and to help you master carbohydrate counting.

TABLE 2-3 How Much Carbohydrate Do You Need?*

	Desire weight loss†	Many older women	Women, older adults	Larger women, older men	Children, teen girls, active women, most men	Teen boys, active men
Calorie level	About 1200	About 1400	About 1600	About 1800	About 2200	About 2800
Calorie range	1200–1500	1300–1600	1400–1700	1600–1900	1800–2300	2200–2800
Carbohydrate grams	180	180	195	210	240	300
Carbohydrate choices	12	12	13	14	16	20
Grains, beans, and starchy vegetables	6	6	6	7	9	11
Vegetables	3	3	3	4	4	5
Fruits	3	3	3	3	3	4
Milk‡	2	2	2–3	2–3	2–3	2–3
Meats	2 (4 oz)	2 (4 oz)	2 (5 oz)	2 (5 oz)	2 (6 oz)	3 (7 oz)
Fats g/servings (based on 30% of calories as fat)	40/4	47/5	54/6	60/7	74/9	93/12

* Chart adapted from *Diabetes Meal Planning Made Easy*, 2nd ed. American Diabetes Association. 2000.
† Some older women and men who are small in stature and sedentary may need to eat no more than 1200 calories to lose weight. At 1200 calories, you may need a vitamin and mineral supplement that provides 100% of the Daily Value to meet your nutrition needs.
‡ Teenagers, young adults to age 24, and women who are pregnant or breastfeeding and adults older than 50 need 1200 mg of calcium each day. Adults younger than 50 need 1000 mg of calcium per day. Each cup of milk or yogurt contains about 300 mg of calcium. Other sources of calcium are calcium-fortified orange juice, other dairy products, and dark green leafy vegetables. If you do not get sufficient calcium from the foods you eat, talk to your health care provider about taking a calcium supplement to meet your requirements for calcium. Each serving of milk is equivalent to about 12 grams of carbohydrate or roughly 1 carbohydrate choice.
   To develop individualized recommendations about the amount of carbohydrate you should eat at meals and snacks, work with a dietitian or diabetes educator with expertise in diabetes and carbohydrate counting.

3

Are You Ready?

Are you ready to measure servings, check lists, count the carbs, check your blood glucose at least 2 times a day, and record the numbers? You'll only have to measure servings and check blood glucose more often for several weeks, or until you can see the pattern to your blood glucose level and what affects it. Carb counting is not hard, but it does take a commitment from you.

Are you ready to:

1. Find a meal planning approach that fits your lifestyle and desire for more flexibility?
You may have tried a variety of meal-planning approaches in the past—the food exchange system, the food guide pyramid, or counting calories. Maybe none of them fit your lifestyle or provide enough flexibility. Carb counting might be the meal planning approach for you.

　　　　　　□ yes　　□ no

2. Find a meal planning approach that helps you achieve better control of your blood glucose levels?
Who doesn't want that? The more carbohydrate you eat, the higher your blood glucose level is going to go. If you know where it's going, you can add exercise or adjust your medication to bring it back down. It makes sense, then, that

if you eat the same amount of carbohydrate at the same meals from day to day, you can control your blood glucose better.

☐ yes ☐ no

3. Learn more about foods and how much carbohydrate is in them?

The three food groups that contain carbohydrates are starches and sugars, fruit, and dairy foods. You will also learn which foods contain protein and fat and why they are important.

☐ yes ☐ no

4. Pay more attention to what you eat and the amount you eat?

You will be able to eat the foods you enjoy, but you need to watch the amounts. Portion control is a skill you will learn and is very helpful in our super-sized society (chapter 7).

☐ yes ☐ no

5. Keep food records that detail the foods, the amount, when you eat, and how much carb is in each food, meal, or snack?

Keeping a record will provide you with a profile of your food choices and the amounts of foods you eat. It will also help you build your own database of carb counts so you don't have to keep looking them up.

☐ yes ☐ no

6. Check blood glucose levels at least two times a day and record the results?

Many things can affect your blood glucose level. If you haven't been checking, you'll need to check it either before or 2 hours after the first bite of the meal for a couple of weeks. This information along with the food information you record gives you a feel for the effect of the carbs you eat on your blood glucose levels.

☐ yes   ☐ no

7. Have the tools to weigh and measure servings—and use them?

You need to measure your servings and get skilled at "guess-timating" the amounts you eat (when you don't have a scale handy), because this is how you count the carbs in the serving. For example, a slice of bread is 1 serving of carbohydrate, 1 carbohydrate choice, or 15 grams of carbohydrate. But this is based on a 1-oz piece of bread. A thicker, heavier slice of bread weighing 3 oz would be 3 carb servings or 45 grams of carbohydrate. So you have to be practiced and aware to correctly estimate the amount of carbohydrate in what you eat.

Do you own or are you willing to purchase the tools for carbohydrate counting—a food scale, measuring cups, and measuring spoons?

Food weighing scale	☐ yes	☐ no
Measuring cups	☐ yes	☐ no
Measuring spoons	☐ yes	☐ no

When you use carb counting, you need to practice, practice, practice to get skilled at portion sizes. And once you are skilled at it, you still need to use the measuring tools occasionally to check that your servings haven't grown over time.

☐ yes   ☐ no

8. Read the Nutrition Facts label on packaged foods to find the carbohydrate content?

☐ yes   ☐ no

9. Spend some time to learn how much carbohydrate you need to eat to keep your blood glucose levels in control? Your food and blood glucose records help you see the effect of carbohydrate foods, which helps you decide how much carbohydrate to eat, how much medication to take, and how much physical activity you need to keep your blood glucose levels within the range you want.

☐ yes   ☐ no

4

How Many Meals and Snacks for You?

You may have been told that people with diabetes need to eat three square meals plus three snacks a day. This advice was true in the past, but times have changed. Today, with more medication options and even some medications that don't cause blood sugar to go too low, you don't necessarily need to eat between-meal snacks. However, you may want to. That's a big difference! Figure out, with your health care provider, how many meals and snacks (if any) are the right number for you to achieve the best control of your blood sugar. This should be based on your habits and schedule, how you manage your diabetes, and your need for flexibility.

A Bit of History

Until 1994 the only category of diabetes pills available for people with type 2 diabetes were sulfonylureas and some types of insulin. Neither allowed much flexibility and could cause blood sugar to fall dangerously low (hypoglycemia). To avoid hypoglycemia people with diabetes on these medications were encouraged to eat 3 meals and 2–3 snacks each day.

A New Day has Dawned

Today a variety of insulin and oral medications are available that work at different times and in different ways. By mixing and matching new medications, we have many more treatment options. Several of the new oral diabetes medications don't even cause hypoglycemia, and a couple of others closely match the quick rise in blood sugar from food and then quickly leave the body (Table 4-1). All of these options allow you and your health care providers to find the medication regimen that most closely matches your diabetes and lifestyle needs. You don't have to eat a set number of meals or snacks at all. You base the decisions about snacks and the size of breakfast, lunch, and dinner on your blood sugar goals and what fits your own lifestyle. Once again, use the feedback from your blood glucose checks to tell you whether you need to adjust your food or your medication, or both.

TABLE 4 - 1 Diabetes Medications and Hypoglycemia	
Diabetes medications that can cause hypoglycemia	Diabetes medications that do not cause hypoglycemia
Sulfonylureas: Amaryl, Glucotrol, Glucotrol XL, DiaBeta, Glynase, Micronase, Orinase, Tolinase, Diabinese, Dymelor **Glucovance** (Glucovance is a combination of metformin and glyburide, a sulfonylurea. The glyburide portion can cause hypoglycemia.) **Meglitinides:** repaglinide (Prandin) **d-phenylalanine:** nateglinide (Starlix) **Insulin**	**Metformin:** Glucophage **Alpha-glucosidase inhibitors:** Precose and Glyset **Glitazones:** Avandia and Actos

There are two relatively new categories of medications that can cause hypoglycemia, but they are less likely to because they act so quickly. In the oral category is meglitinides and the two available pills are repaglinide (Prandin) and nateglinide (Starlix). Meglitinides are taken just before you eat, and they help the pancreas quickly produce insulin to help lower the blood sugar rise that occurs from the carbohydrate you eat. They work quickly and leave the body quickly. As long as the meal is sufficient to match the amount of medication, the risk of hypoglycemia is small. In the insulin category, two brands of rapid-acting insulin are now available: lispro (Humalog) and aspart (Novolog). The rapid-acting insulin also works with the rise in blood sugar from a meal. It starts working within 5–15 minutes and peaks in 45–90 minutes. It clears your system within 3 hours. Again the carb content of the meal must be appropriate for the amount of insulin you're taking. But with their quick action, you don't need to be a slave to snacking to prevent hypoglycemia several hours later.

How Many Meals and Snacks Do You Eat?

You are most likely to get the best control of blood sugar if you eat about the same amount of carbohydrate at the same meals and snacks from day to day. That's particularly true if you don't adjust the amount of medication you take for the amount of carbohydrate you eat. However, for most people this plan just doesn't mesh with real life. Very few people eat planned meals from day to day. Most Americans tend to eat breakfast—if they eat breakfast—as they're flying out the door or in the car. Lunch is usually a quick meal but larger than breakfast and dinner. Dinner is typically the largest meal of the day. If the way you eat looks like this, then your health care providers need to take this into account when they prescribe types and amounts of diabetes medications.

A word to the wise: Let your health care provider know as much about your eating style and daily schedule as you can. Don't let them prescribe medications for you based on a pretend 9-to-5 lifestyle that simply isn't so. Let them know whether you prefer 3-meals and 2-snacks or 3-meals and no snacks. Tell them the times you eat meals or snacks. This information is helpful because some diabetes medications have an onset, peak, and duration of action. The action curve needs to be in synch with when you eat. Help your health care provider learn enough about you to set your medication plan around your real eating habits, instead of setting up your medication schedule and then you have to eat to meet the action of the meds.

Even if you are not asked to keep a food diary, you might want to do so anyway. You may not know what your real eating habits are. A record gives information about your food choices and lifestyle that you can discuss with your health care provider. Let your provider know if you often have hypoglycemia, feel hungry, or are gaining weight. These could be signs that your diabetes medication is not matching well with your lifestyle. Also, the records of your blood sugar checks are the best way for you to know whether your blood sugar is under control. Remember, there are a variety of diabetes medications to design a diabetes plan that is flexible enough to fit your lifestyle.

To snack or not?

Here are several points to consider when deciding how many meals and snacks are right for you.

1. Would you rather have 6 small meals or 3 larger meals a day?

2. Do you enjoy snacks at certain times of the day or do you feel snacks are just a bother?
3. If you like to snack, what time(s) of the day do you want a snack?
4. Do you feel that you need snacks for good nutrition or to better manage your blood sugar?

What foods make good snacks?

There are healthy and not-so-healthy snacks available today. The ideal snack is fresh, convenient to purchase or carry, and easy to eat. A few healthy, convenient snacks are: fruit, fruit juice, yogurt, milk, popcorn, pretzels, and crackers to name a few. Unfortunately these may not be as available as the not-so-healthy snacks that are high in calories, fat, and sodium, such as potato and corn chips, cookies, candy, and ice cream. To eat healthy snacks you need to plan ahead—for example to cut up the raw veggies you want to take to work. The benefit of planning is that you get a snack packed with fiber, vitamins, and minerals. Appendix 1 has carb counts for various foods that you might choose for healthy snacks.

Should you have fruit or fruit juice for a snack?

Yes, because most Americans don't eat enough fruit. Some people with diabetes have been told not to eat fruit or fruit juice as a snack because they cause a quick rise in blood sugar. But research shows that most sources of carbohydrate raise blood sugar to about the same level in about the same amount of time. Fruit and fruit juice are no exception. In fact, some studies have shown that fruit raises blood sugar more slowly than some other carbohydrates because it is about 50% fructose. So if you need to eat more fruit to improve your diet and the only way you can fit it in is for snacks, try it. Then a couple of times check your blood sugar 2 hours later to see how high it rises. If it is too high, then try eating fruit with a meal instead.

Should snacks contain carbohydrate and protein?

For years people have been taught that between-meal snacks and especially bedtime snacks, should contain carbohydrate and protein—crackers and cheese or peanut butter, half a turkey or roast beef sandwich, or graham crackers and milk. The thought was that protein is a longer-lasting source of energy, and it would keep blood sugar levels up longer to prevent hypoglycemia. Some studies do show that protein helps to reduce the rise in blood sugar after a meal or snack, so you may want to continue these protein-carb snacks if your records show that this is true for you. This particularly might be true during the night. If you don't find that protein in the snack helps you keep your blood sugar in control and that you'd rather eat your protein at meals, talk to your health care providers about adjusting your diabetes plan. See chapter 6.

Are diabetes snack products beneficial?

If you've recently cruised the aisles of supermarkets or skimmed the pages of magazines, you know there are snack bars and drinks designed just for people with diabetes. These products may tout their ability to improve blood glucose control or reduce the risk of nighttime hypoglycemia. Several contain odd sounding ingredients and some pack in lots of vitamins and minerals. Should you spend your hard-earned dollar on these products?

There are pluses. These bars and drinks offer a quick and easy choice that may be healthier than your current snacks because they contain essential vitamins and minerals. These products are handy for on-the-run meals or used before, during, or after exercise. A few small studies show that beyond just providing calories and vitamins and minerals, the bars and drinks may slow down and lower the rise of blood glucose a few hours after consumption. This effect is due either to a carbohydrate-based ingredient in several products or to the ratio of nutrients.

There are minuses. These products can be expensive. Perhaps a more economical choice would be healthy snack foods and a vitamin and mineral supplement. Also, if you eat these foods regularly, and they lower your blood glucose levels, you'll need to work with your health provider to learn how to adjust your diabetes medicine and fit these products into your eating plan.

If you find one or more of these diabetes products works well for you, you and your health care provider need to fit them into your eating plan. Don't eat them as extras. They have calories. A word of caution: use them only to prevent low blood glucose (hypoglycemia), not to treat it. The slower-acting carbohydrates won't bring blood glucose up as fast as regular carbohydrate-containing foods do. Lastly, don't think of these as a quick fix to blood glucose control, but just as a potential aid.

Meet Matt

Matt is 50 years old and was diagnosed with type 2 diabetes 5 years ago. He takes metformin twice a day—before breakfast and before dinner. He just recently learned that he is not at risk for developing low blood sugar while taking metformin. Matt has to be at work at 5 a.m. and doesn't get time to eat lunch till 12 noon, and then he eats his evening meal around 7 p.m. He eats two snacks a day: one snack between breakfast and lunch and the other between lunch and dinner. He doesn't eat a nighttime snack because he goes to bed around 9 p.m. Matt wanted to continue to eat two snacks a day because the time between his meals was too long to go without food. Though Matt didn't need to eat snacks to prevent hypoglycemia, he chose to eat snacks because it fits best with his wants and nutrition needs.

Meet Sue

Sue is 35 years old and has had type 1 diabetes for 10 years. She has always had to work hard to control her weight. Sue has been on two injections of insulin a day for many years.

She takes an intermediate-acting insulin (NPH) and regular insulin before breakfast and before dinner. She has been encouraged to eat a mid-afternoon and a bedtime snack to keep her blood sugar from dipping too low. She is a traveling salesperson for a large food service company. She does not always get lunch or a mid-afternoon snack on time, and she gets shaky and sweaty, due to hypoglycemia. She then panics and over-treats the low blood sugars with high calorie foods such as ice cream or chocolate. Sue would prefer not to snack because it is inconvenient in her job and hinders maintaining her weight. After reading an article about rapid-acting insulin, she approached her doctor with the article, a one-week food diary, and her blood sugar records.

She noted that she is tired of having to snack to keep her blood sugar up, and she pointed to the time constraints of her job and daily schedule. She asked if an insulin regimen with rapid-acting insulin was for her. Her doctor said, "Let's give it a try." She began taking rapid-acting insulin before breakfast along with NPH insulin. Then she took rapid-acting insulin before dinner and NPH before bed. Her doctor sent her to a dietitian to learn more about carb counting.

After a few weeks of checking her blood sugars, she realized her numbers were up before lunch and about two hours after lunch. Her doctor suggested she begin taking some rapid-acting insulin before lunch as well to bring those numbers closer to her target range. For convenience Sue learned how to use an insulin pen. Slowly but surely, Sue's blood sugar was getting into better control, and best yet, she didn't have to be bothered with between-meal snacks. She began to lose one pound every few weeks.

5

Begin Counting

To begin carb counting you need to get to know yourself better. That is your eating habits—what, when, and how much you eat. The best way to accomplish this is to keep records of your current food habits—a food diary. Look at the flow of your average day. Maybe you'll see that you start the day with the same breakfast at the same time, but lunch and dinner are never even close to similar times. Or maybe you'll learn that you follow a pretty tight schedule during the week, but on the weekends your schedule changes dramatically. Or maybe your meal times are different everyday.

To be successful with basic carbohydrate counting, you'll need to figure out how much carbohydrate you eat and when—on most days. Eating similar amounts of carb on a fairly regular schedule helps you control your blood sugar levels. Keep good *and honest* records. It's the only way you can trust your results and put them to good use to control your blood glucose.

Step 1: Keep Food Records

Begin keeping a food diary by writing down the foods you eat at breakfast, lunch, and dinner. Don't forget to include snacks and nibbles. Yes, crumbs do count! Keep these records for a full week including the weekend. Beyond recording the food, write down the amount you eat as well. If it would help to dust off the measuring cups and spoons to get more accurate quantities, do so. The more accurate you can be, the more helpful your food records will be to you and to your health care provider. Remember, it's not just what you eat, but the all-important "size" of your serving as well. You can design and use a food record like the ones shown in Table 5-1.

Step 2: Find the Foods with Carbohydrate

Now that you have one week of your food diary completed, go through and circle the foods that contain any carbohydrate (Table 5-2 on pages 42–43). Don't forget that dairy foods, fruits, and desserts contain carb and that you might also pick up a few grams from fat-free salad dressing. This helps you learn to identify the foods you typically eat and which ones contain carbohydrates.

Step 3: Figure How Much Carb You Eat

Now, figure how many grams (g) of carbohydrate you eat at each meal. To do this use the list of foods in Appendix 1 or in other carb counting resources listed in Appendix 3. Fill in the grams of carb as we've done in Table 5-3. Next add up the totals for each meal and snack. If you plan to use carb choices rather than carb grams, remember that each carb choice has 15 grams of carbohydrate.

Step 4: Sit Back and Observe

Are you eating the same amount of carbs at your breakfasts, lunches, dinners, and snacks? In the two days of example records, the carbs in the breakfasts vary from 75 to 102 grams. And the times at which breakfast is eaten are very different, too. One day breakfast is at 7 a.m. and the next it's at 9 a.m. As you have already learned, varying the amount of carb and the timing of breakfast will make it

TABLE 5-1   Food Diary

Breakfast
Time: 7 a.m.

Food	Amount
Blueberry bagel	1 whole
Light cream cheese	2 Tbsp
Strawberries	1 cup sliced

Lunch
Time: 12 noon

Food	Amount
Thin crust cheese pizza	3 14" slices
Garden salad	1 1/2 cups
Thousand Island dressing	2 T
Frozen yogurt cone	1 small

Dinner
Time: 6:30 p.m.

Food	Amount
Grilled chicken	5 oz cooked
Barbecue sauce	2 T
Long grain rice casserole	1 cup
Corn on the cob	1 large
Margarine	2 T
Applesauce (no sugar added)	1 cup

Snack
Time: 9 p.m.

Food	Amount
Oatmeal raisin cookie	1 large

TABLE 5 - 1 Food Diary (continued)

Tuesday

Breakfast
Time: 9 a.m.

Food	Amount
Raisin bran muffin	1
Orange juice	8 oz
Milk, fat free	8 oz

Lunch
Time: 12:30 p.m.

Food	Amount
Chicken pot pie	8 oz
Dinner roll	1
Apple, medium	6 oz

Dinner
Time: 7:45 p.m.

Food	Amount
Spaghetti	2 cups
Meat sauce	3/4 cup
Parmesan cheese	2 Tbsp
Green salad	1 cup
Fat-free french	2 Tbsp

Snack
Time: 10:30 p.m.

Food	Amount
Light ice cream	1 cup
Blueberries	1/2 cup

TABLE 5-2 Food Diary

Monday

Breakfast
Time: 7 a.m.

Food	Amount
Blueberry bagel	1 whole
Light cream cheese	2 Tbsp
Strawberries	1 cup sliced

Lunch
Time: 12 noon

Food	Amount
Thin crust cheese pizza	3 14" slices
Garden salad	1 1/2 cups
Thousand island dressing	2 Tbsp
Frozen yogurt cone	1 small

Dinner
Time: 6:30 p.m.

Food	Amount
Grilled chicken	5 oz cooked
Barbecue sauce	2 Tbsp
Long grain rice casserole	1 cup
Corn on the cob	1 large
Margarine	2 Tbsp
Applesauce (no sugar added)	1 cup

Snack
Time: 9 p.m.

Food	Amount
Oatmeal raisin cookie	1 large

TABLE 5-2 Food Diary (continued)

Tuesday

Breakfast
Time: 9 a.m.

Food	Amount
Raisin bran muffin	1
Orange juice	8 oz
Milk, fat free	8 oz

Lunch
Time: 12:30 p.m.

Food	Amount
Chicken pot pie	8 oz
Dinner roll	1
Apple, medium	6 oz

Dinner
Time: 7:45 p.m.

Food	Amount
Spaghetti	2 cups
Meat sauce	3/4 cup
Parmesan cheese	2 Tbsp
Green salad	1 cup
Fat-free French	2 Tbsp

Snack
Time: 10:30 p.m.

Food	Amount
Light ice cream	1 cup
Blueberries	1/2 cup

TABLE 5-3 Food Diary

Monday

Breakfast
Time: 7 a.m.

Food	Amount	Carb grams
Blueberry bagel	1 whole	61
Light cream cheese	2 Tbsp	2
Strawberries	1 cup sliced	12
		Total carb: 75

Lunch
Time: 12 noon

Food	Amount	Carb grams
Thin crust cheese pizza	3 14" slices	66
Garden salad	1 1/2 cups	0
Thousand island dressing	2 Tbsp	3
Frozen yogurt cone	1 small	23
		Total carb: 92

Dinner
Time: 6:30 p.m.

Food	Amount	Carb grams
Grilled chicken	5 oz cooked	0
Barbecue sauce	2 Tbsp	4
Long grain rice casserole	1 cup	41
Corn on the cob	1 large	32
Margarine	2 Tbsp	0
Applesauce (no sugar added)	1 cup	30
		Total carb: 107

Snack
Time: 9 p.m.

Food	Amount	Carb grams
Oatmeal raisin cookie	1 large	34
		Total carb: 34

TABLE 5-3 Food Diary (continued)

Tuesday

Breakfast
Time: 9 a.m.

Food	Amount	Carb grams
Raisin bran muffin	1	60
Orange juice	8 oz	30
Milk, fat free	8 oz	12
		Total carb: 102

Lunch
Time: 12:30 p.m.

Food	Amount	Carb grams
Chicken pot pie	8 oz	35
Dinner roll	1	16
Apple, medium	6 oz	20
		Total carb: 71

Dinner
Time: 7:45 p.m.

Food	Amount	Carb grams
Spaghetti	2 cups	60
Meat sauce	3/4 cup	16
Parmesan cheese	2 Tbsp	0
Green salad	1 cup	0
Fat-free french	2 Tbsp	12
		Total carb: 88

Snack
Time: 10:30 p.m.

Food	Amount	Carb grams
Light ice cream	1 cup	40
Blueberries	1/2 cup	10
		Total carb: 50

difficult to control blood sugar levels. That's particularly true if you, like most people, take the same amount of diabetes medicine each day. Then especially, you need to keep the amount of carbohydrate you eat at meals and snacks fairly consistent to achieve a steady pattern in your blood sugar levels (see page 18).

Step 5: Get Familiar with Carb Counts

We all tend to eat similar foods on most days. Sure, once in a while we eat an ethnic meal in a restaurant or we try a new recipe, but the rest of the time we eat the same foods over and over. This actually makes carb counting easier—once you learn the carb counts of the foods you regularly eat. You can start to create your own "database" of carb counts. Keep it in a notebook or in a computer file—whatever works best for you (Table 5-4). Look at the Nutrition Facts panels of foods in your pantry, freezer, and refrigerator, and check out the carb count. If you regularly eat pizza or sub sandwiches in restaurants, see if the restaurant can

TABLE 5-4 Sample Personal Database Record		
Food	Serving (amount I eat)	Grams of carbohydrate
Bagel (Dunkin' Donuts)— pumpernickel	1	70
Grandma Grace's apple cobbler	3/4 cup	35 (from recipe analysis)
Domino's cheese pizza with onions and mushrooms— hand tossed	2 14" pieces	45
Healthy Choice Ginger Chicken Hunan	1 entree	59
Weight Watcher's Garden Lasagna	1 entree	30

provide you with nutrition information or use one of the resources in Appendix 3.

Step 6: How Much Carb Should You Eat?

Now you have gotten a picture of how much carbohydrate you eat at your meals and snacks. Look at the chart on page 25 to determine the grams of carb or carb choices you need based on your age, sex, and level of activity. Compare your records to this chart and ask yourself: are you eating too much, too little, or just the right amount of carb for you? At this point you might want to consult with your health care provider or set up a visit with a dietitian with expertise in carb counting to help you design a carb counting plan.

Step 7: Match Up What You Eat with Blood Sugar Records

The next step is to match your food records with your blood sugar records. Learning how your meals and certain foods affect your blood sugar will help you and your health care provider fine-tune your diabetes management plan. Unfortunately most of the blood sugar records that come with your glucose meter or other diabetes supplies don't provide much room for you to record what you eat and how much carb you eat. We encourage you to try the record form in Appendix 3. You might want to change the form here and there to fit your needs. Table 5-5 is a sample form.

The recording form provides room to record:

- the timing of your meals and snacks

- the type and dose of your diabetes medications

- the food you eat including the amount and the grams of carb or carb choices

- the results of your blood sugar checks with a note of the time of the check

TABLE 5-5 Carbohydrate Counting and Blood Glucose Results Record

Day/Date: *Tuesday, June 3*

Time/ meal	Diabetes medicines		Food		Carb grams
	Type	**Amount**	**Type**	**Amount**	
6:45 a.m./	NPH	12u			
	R	5u			
7 a.m./b'fast			Shredded Wheat 'n Bran with	1/2 cup	20
			Cheerios	3/4 cup	17
			Milk	1 cup	12
			Banana	1 medium	20
					Total 69
12:30 p.m.			Sub sandwich– 12" turkey, ham, cheese, lettuce, tomato, onions, pickles, mustard	1	92
			Pretzels	2 1/2 oz bag	34
					Total 126
5:00 p.m./Snack			Apple	8 oz/1 large	30
7:15 p.m.	NPH	9u			
	R	4u			
Dinner			Macaroni and cheese, prepared with sliced turkey sausage	2 cups	98
			Broccoli, steamed	1 cup	8
			Fruit cup	3/4 cup	22
					Total 128

Notes about day:
Went for a walk after dinner.
Blood sugar has gotten low right before bed several times recently.

				Blood glucose results			
Fasting/ before b'fast/ time	**After b'fast/ time**	**Before lunch/ time**	**After lunch/ time**	**Before dinner/ time**	**After dinner/ time**	**Before bed/ time**	**Other/ time**
92/ 6:30	210/ 8:45 a.m.						
		89/ 12:30	154/ 2:00				
				126/ 7:00 p.m.	205/ 9:00 p.m.		Checked at 11 p.m., felt low, BS = 65

■ an "other" column to record the type and amount of your physical activity, your daily schedule, emotions or stressful situations, or other reasons why your blood sugar results might have been different than expected. You can also record information about activity, emotions, and general observations under "notes."

Recording More Details

Diabetes medications

Some people with diabetes take no medication, some people take one or more pills, and some people take insulin or a combination of pills and insulin. It is this wonderful variety of medications that provides the many options with which to control blood sugar. Know the type of diabetes medication you take. Know when to take it, understand how it works to help control blood sugar, and how the medication works in conjunction with the carb you eat to control your blood sugar. Record type, dose, and timing of each medication. Having this information recorded helps you interpret your blood sugar results.

Table 5-6 lists the diabetes medications available today. There will be even more in the future. Find the diabetes medication(s) that you take to learn more about them.

Checking Blood Sugar

To gain the best understanding of the ups and downs of your blood sugar in response to food, activity, stress, and other things in your life, check your blood glucose at various times of the day. And most importantly, record the results. If you don't record the results, the data you could learn from is lost. Another section on the example form is for after-meal blood sugar checks. As you are learning, these results are very important, but most commercial record books don't provide space for these results. After-meal

TABLE 5 - 6 Diabetes Medications

Category	Generic and brand name of medication	Action to control blood glucose	Side effects	Carbohydrate counting
Sulfonylureas	Chlorpropamide (Diabinese) Tolazamide (Tolinase) Tolbutamide (Orinase) Glipizide (Glucotrol, Glucotrol XL) Glyburide (Glynase, DiaBeta, Micronase) Glimepiride (Amaryl)	Helps the pancreas make more insulin. Usually take before a meal once or twice a day. Can combine with metformin, alpha glucosidase inhibitors, glitazones, or insulin.	Could cause hypoglycemia and weight gain.	Carbohydrate needs to be similar at meals and snacks.
Meglitinides	Repaglinide (Prandin)	Helps pancreas quickly produce insulin to lower blood sugar after eating. Take before meals.	Can cause hypoglycemia if medication is taken but you don't eat or only eat a small amount.	Best if carb content of meals is similar, however you can learn to adjust the amount of medication for the amount of food you eat at the meal.
D-phenylalanine	Nateglinides (Starlix)		Same as the meglitinides	

TABLE 5 - 6 Diabetes Medications (continued)

Category	Generic and brand name of medication	Action to control blood glucose	Side effects	Carbohydrate counting
Biguanide	Metformin (Glucophage, Glucophage XR)	Lowers blood glucose by decreasing liver production of glucose. Can combine with sulfonylureas, glitazones, alpha-glucosidase inhibitors, or insulin.	Upset stomach; may lose a few pounds when start taking; do not take if you have kidney or liver disease. Do not take pill if you drink alcohol daily. Does not cause hypoglycemia.	Best if carb content of meals is similar.
Biguanide/ sulfonylureas combination	Glucovance (combination of metformin and glyburide)	Action of biguanide and sulfonylurea.	Can cause hypoglycemia.	Best if carb content of meals is similar.
Glitazones	Rosiglitazone (Avandia) Pioglitazone (Actos)	Helps sensitize your body's tissues to better use the insulin you make. Can combine with sulfonylureas, alpha-glucosidase inhibitors, metformin, or insulin.	Not to be used if you have liver problems. It can interfere with the working of birth control pills. Does not cause hypoglycemia. Can cause weight gain.	Best if carb content of meals is similar.

Alpha-glucosidase inhibitors	Acarbose (Precose) Miglitol (Glyset)	Slows the breakdown of carbohydrates in the food you eat. Reduces the blood glucose rise after the meal.	Gas, bloating; do not use if there is no carbohydrate in the meal. Does not cause hypoglycemia.	Best if carb content of meals is similar.
Insulin	Rapid-acting: lispro, aspart Short-acting: regular Intermediate-acting: NPH, Lente Long-acting: Ultralente, glargine (Lantus) Premixed combinations: 70/30, 50/50 (NPH and regular) 75/25 (NPH and lispro)	Lowers blood sugar by putting insulin into the body.	Can cause hypoglycemia and weight gain.	Carb content of meals can vary if you learn to adjust insulin based on your insulin: carbohydrate ratio.

(1 1/2 to 2 hours after the time you begin eating) blood sugar checks help you see the impact of the carbohydrate you ate at that meal. Your blood sugar needs to be in target range both before meals and after. The chart on page 7 gives you the normal ranges of blood glucose so you can see where yours are in relation to them.

Now don't be alarmed, you don't need to check your blood sugar seven times a day! To observe the ups and downs in your blood sugar, yet avoid feeling like a human pincushion, set up a rotating blood sugar checking pattern. Check your blood glucose 2 times a day at different times on different days. In just a few days, you'll have results from around the clock.

Here's a 4-day sample pattern with 2 checks a day.

	Fasting	1–2 hrs after breakfast	Before lunch	1–2 hrs after lunch	Before dinner	1–2 hrs after dinner	Bed	Other
Day 1	■	■						
Day 2			■	■				
Day 3					■	■		
Day 4	■						■	

Here's a 7-day pattern with 2 checks a day: one fasting and the other at different times each day. You check 1–2 hours after the time you start to eat.

	Fasting	1–2 hrs after breakfast	Before lunch	1–2 hrs after lunch	Before dinner	1–2 hrs after dinner	Bed	Other
Day 1	■	■						
Day 2	■		■					
Day 3	■			■				
Day 4	■				■			
Day 5	■					■		
Day 6	■						■	
Day 7	■							■

There are many patterns to chose from. Your health care provider can suggest one to help you focus on a particular question to be answered.

Physical Activity

In almost all cases, being physically active lowers blood sugar. Being physically active is an important part of managing your diabetes as well as an important part of staying healthy and controlling blood lipids and blood pressure. If you are not physically active, think about what you are willing to start doing. Perhaps it's a 20-minute walk 2 times a week or 15 minutes on your stationary bike 3 times a week or simply some more housework or gardening. Don't forget—any physical activity helps!

Use the "other" column or the "notes" section at the bottom to record the type and amount of physical activity you do and when you do them.

Emotions, Stress, Illness, and Unusual Situations

We know that changes in day-to-day events can and do affect blood sugar levels. It's important to record information about your emotions and stressful situations. Illness, medical tests, or surgery can impact your blood sugar. And so can a deadline at work or a heated argument, even if you're just a bystander. It's also important to record positive emotions and situations, too. For example, vacations might be a positive situation, however, you eat differently and at different times. You may be well yourself, but you have a sick child or a family emergency. Women should note menstrual periods on the form as well. The various phases of the menstrual cycle, including the hormonal surges of adolescence and menopause, can impact blood sugar levels. You can use the "other" column or "notes" at the bottom for recording these events.

Meet Jane

Jane is a 45-year-old schoolteacher who was recently diagnosed with type 2 diabetes. She takes 500 mg of Glucophage before breakfast and dinner. She feels she gets enough physical activity at work. She is interested in carb counting as a way to keep her blood sugar in control, but also have flexibility with the food choices she makes.

She checks her blood sugar when she gets up and does a second check at various times before and after meals. One day she checks after lunch and the next day after dinner but always within 1–2 hours after she starts eating. Her blood sugars after lunch are 140–175, within her target range after meals. But the ones after dinner are in the 200–230 range, and she is concerned about this. She looks at the amount of carbs she eats—about 60 grams at lunch and 110 grams at dinner. She sees that she is not active when she gets home. She fixes dinner and watches her favorite TV shows. But after lunch, she is teaching and on her feet and moving for 3 more hours.

Keeping records helped Jane learn how the amount of carbs she eats and her activity level has an effect on her blood sugar. She realizes she needs to balance the amount of carb she eats each day by eating more at lunch when she is active and less in the evening. She and the dietitian she is working with set a goal of 60–75 grams of carb at lunch and dinner.

You can see Jane's record in Table 5-7 on the next two pages.

TABLE 5-7 Carbohydrate Counting and Blood Glucose Results Record

Day/Date: *Tuesday, January 23*

Time/ meal	Diabetes medicines		Food		Carb count (choices/ grams)
	Type	Amount	Type	Amount	
6:00 a.m./ 6:15 a.m./ B'fast	Gluco- phage	500 mg			
			Frozen waffles	2	29
			Maple syrup	2 Tbsp	26
			Raspberries	1/2 cup	8
			Yogurt with fruit, nonfat with low- cal sweetener	1/2 cup	10
					Total 73
12:30 p.m./ Lunch			Chunky split pea and ham soup	1 11-oz can	33
			Ritz crackers	5	9
			Pear	1 6 oz	22
					Total 64
6:00 p.m./ Dinner	Gluco- phage	500 mg	Pork chop—baked	3 oz	0
			Mashed potatoes	1 cup	33
			with butter	1 tsp	0
			Green peas	1/2 cup	15
			Dinner roll	1	15
			with butter	1 tsp	0
			Apple pie	1/8 9" pie	43
					Total 106

Notes about day:
On my feet and moving while teaching after lunch for 3 hours.

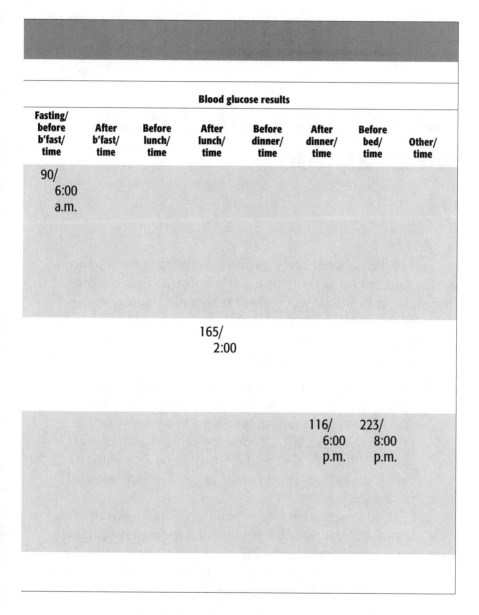

Blood glucose results

Fasting/ before b'fast/ time	After b'fast/ time	Before lunch/ time	After lunch/ time	Before dinner/ time	After dinner/ time	Before bed/ time	Other/ time
90/ 6:00 a.m.							
			165/ 2:00				
					116/ 6:00 p.m.	223/ 8:00 p.m.	

6

Count Foods with Protein and Fat, Too

T rue, the focus of carbohydrate counting is on the foods that contain carbohydrate. It's also true that the protein and fat in foods, when you eat them in the recommended amounts, have very little effect on your blood glucose levels. But, you cannot ignore foods that contain protein and fat. Here are some good reasons why:

1. Protein and fat have calories. So, protein and fat might not impact your blood glucose levels much, but if you eat too much, they can add to your waistline. Examples of high-fat foods are salad dressings, margarine, mayonnaise, and cream cheese. Some foods are high in both protein and fat, such as cheese and sausage.

2. Fat and protein in your meal may slow down the rise in blood glucose. When you eat a meal that is higher in protein than usual, for example, you enjoy an 8-oz steak or prime rib, your blood glucose might rise more slowly than you expect. Also, when you eat a meal that is higher in fat than usual, for example, fried chicken, mashed potatoes, and gravy followed by a piece of cheesecake for dessert, your blood glucose might rise more slowly and peak later than you expect. You need to learn to account for these differences.

3. Too much protein, especially animal protein, and too much fat, especially saturated fat, are not healthy—for anyone.

The Purpose of Protein and Fat

Our bodies need some protein to build muscles. Protein is made up of amino acids that the body needs in order to work. Interestingly, several amino acids can be converted into glucose. This glucose can enter the bloodstream and be used for energy.

Our bodies also need some fat, but only a small amount. Fat carries the fat-soluble vitamins A, D, E, and K. A couple of so-called "essential" fats must be in the foods you eat because the body can't make them. Fats supply energy, cushion the body's vital organs, and provide insulation to keep us warm. Also, fat is well known for making food taste good.

Which foods contain protein?

Many people would answer "red meat, poultry, and seafood." But actually protein turns up in other food groups, too. Red meat, poultry, seafood, eggs, and cheese are sources of protein, but they have varying amounts of fat. Foods from other food groups contain protein but it's mixed up with carbohydrate—dried beans and peas, grains, and vegetables. Then there are nuts. They contain protein, but they are in the fat food group because most of their calories come from fat. Table 6-1 shows the food groups that contain protein.

Which foods contain fat?

Some foods are just about 100% fat, such as butter, margarine, or regular salad dressing. They are often added to other foods to make them taste better. You might call these "added fats." Plenty of foods contain zero fat, such as

TABLE 6-1 Nutrients in Foods

Food group	Serving†	Nutrients* Carbohydrate (g) 4 calories/g	Protein (g) 4 calories/g	Fat (g) 9 calories/g
Bread	1 slice	15	3	0
Cereal, dry	1 oz	15	3	‡
Cereal, cooked	1/2 cup	15	3	‡
Pasta	1/2 cup	15	3	‡
Starchy vegetable	1/3 to 1/2 cup	15	3	0
Fruit, fresh	1 medium piece	15	0	0
Fruit juice	1/3 to 1/2 cup	15	0	0
Fruit, canned, no sugar added	1/2 cup	15	0	0
Vegetables	1/2 cup cooked	5	0	0
Vegetable	1 cup raw	5	0	0
Milk, fat free	1 cup	12	8	0
Yogurt, plain, nonfat	3/4 cup	12	8	0
Sugary foods	1 serving	Varies	Varies	Varies
Sweets	1 serving	Varies	Varies	Varies
Meats	3 oz cooked	0	21	Varies
Fats—margarine, mayonnaise, oil	1 tsp	0	0	5

* Alcohol contains 7 calories per gram and is considered a nutrient.
† Servings are according to servings in *Exchange Lists for Meal Planning* published by ADA and The American Dietetic Association, 1995.
‡ Depends on cereal or the grain.

pasta, broccoli, and lettuce—that is until you add fat when you cook them or at the table. Other foods contain some, but not all, of their calories as fat, such as meats, cheese, nuts, whole-milk dairy foods, and most desserts. You might call these "attached fats," where fat is naturally part of the food. Table 6-1 shows the food groups that contain fat.

Fats are actually combinations of different types of fatty acids. In foods, the fat is made up of varying amounts of three types of fat—saturated fat, polyunsaturated fat, and monounsaturated fat. Here are some examples of the three types of fat.

MONOUNSATURATED FATS (Most beneficial)

- Oils (canola, olive, peanut)
- Olives
- Nuts
- Peanut butter

POLYUNSATURATED FATS

- Margarine
- Mayonnaise
- Oils (corn, safflower, soybean)

SATURATED FATS (most important to limit)

- Bacon
- Butter
- Cream cheese
- Sour cream

What does protein do to blood glucose?

For many years it was thought that 50% of the protein we ate was converted into glucose and that protein just raised blood glucose more slowly than carbohydrate. This theory encouraged health professionals to teach people with diabetes to always eat protein in combination with carbohydrate at meals and snacks. Newer research questions whether this is always true. Recent research shows that protein stimulates the production of some insulin in people with type 2 diabetes and that this small rise in insulin actually lowers blood glucose. In people with type 1 diabetes, protein has little effect on blood glucose, unless very large portions are eaten. Large portions of protein can increase blood glucose and cause a need for more insulin or other diabetes medication.

So, what's the advice about protein today? Monitor your blood glucose and see what works best for you. Some people feel they do better with some protein at each meal. Other people feel that protein in a bedtime snack is helpful. Still others don't think the added protein makes a difference. Also, it can be difficult to spread the small amount of protein recommended in most meal plans across meals and snacks.

It is true that a high-protein meal—which often is both a high-protein and high-fat meal—may delay the rise of blood glucose. In other words, the high amount of protein and fat slow down the rise of blood glucose from the carbohydrate in the meal. This may be due, in part, to a delay in stomach emptying. If you are used to eating a 3–4-oz serving of meat at dinner and you treat yourself to an 8-oz sirloin, you might find that when you check your blood glucose level 2 hours later, it's not as high as you thought it would be. Then if you check it 3–4 hours later, when you thought it would be headed down, it is higher than you expected. There are various ways to manage this situation (chapter 12), but keep in mind that it is healthiest to eat small amounts of protein and fat.

Meet Jan

Jan is a person with type 1 diabetes. She takes 3 shots of insulin a day—one shot of glargine (Lantus) at bedtime, and rapid-acting lispro before meals (see Table 6-2). She has had the experience of eating a meal high in protein and fat and finding that her blood sugar is not as high as she expected

TABLE 6-2 Jan's Record: High-Protein, High-Fat Meal (Person with type 1 diabetes)

Day/Date: *Tuesday, January 23*

Time/meal	Diabetes medicines		Food		Carb count (choices/grams)	Before dinner (7 p.m.)	Blood glucose results 2 hours (9 p.m.)	3 hours (10 p.m.)	Bedtime (11 p.m.)
	Type	Amount	Type	Amount					
7 p.m.	Humalog	6 units	Sirloin steak	8 oz		107	155	261	143
			Baked potato with	6 oz	2/30 g				
			Sour cream	2 T					
			Butter	2 t					
			Salad bar with	1 trip	2/30 g				
			Thousand island dressing	3 T	0.5/7 g				
			Dinner roll	1 medium	1/15 g				
			Butter	1 t					
			Strawberry shortcake	1/2 portion	2/35 g				
			Total		8/117 g				

2 hours after she started eating. This evening she decided that she was going to check her blood sugar more often to determine the effect of a high protein and fat meal. She'll take them to her diabetes care provider to talk about taking more rapid-acting insulin before a meal that is larger than usual or even taking the insulin in the middle or at the end of the meal to better control the after-meal blood sugar level.

Meet Eric   Eric has type 2 diabetes, is overweight, and is quite insulin resistant. He takes Glucophage before breakfast and dinner and takes Prandin, a rapid-acting diabetes pill, before his three meals. He decided to check his blood sugar levels a number of times after eating a rather high protein and fat meal. He wanted to learn what this type of meal and foods did to his blood sugar (Table 6-3). With his chart in hand, he talked to his diabetes care provider about the possibility of increasing his dose of Prandin for a meal like this. However, he recognizes very well that doing this on a regular basis would probably make him gain weight and not do much for his arteries either.

It is also known that certain foods, pizza being one of them, can have a delayed and somewhat unpredictable effect on blood sugar levels (Table 6-4).

It is important to note that the impact of eating larger than usual amounts of protein and fat varies from person to person and varies according to each person's diabetes management plan. The best advice is to monitor your blood glucose several times in the hours after the meal when you eat meals or foods that are higher in protein and fat. For instance, you might want to check your blood glucose both 2 hours and 3 hours after the meal rather than just 2 hours after. At 2 hours you might not have seen the full impact of the meal on your blood glucose level. Learn how your body responds to these meals, so you can determine a plan to manage them.

Day/Date: *Tuesday, January 23*

| Time/ meal | Diabetes medicines | | Food | | Carb count (choices/ grams) | Blood glucose results | | | | |
	Type	Amount	Type	Amount		Before dinner (7 p.m.)	2 hours (9 p.m.)	3 hours (10 p.m.)	Bedtime (11 p.m.)	
7 p.m.	Glucophage	850 mg	Sirloin steak	8 oz		147	198	280	223	
			Baked potato with	6 oz	2/30 g					
			Sour cream	2 T						
			Butter	2 t						
			Salad bar with	1 trip	2/30 g					
			Thousand island dressing	3 T	0.5/7 g					
			Dinner roll	1 medium	1/15 g					
			Butter	1 t						
			Strawberry shortcake	1/2 portion	2/35 g					
			Total		8/117 g					

TABLE 6-4 Sample Record: Effect of Pizza on Blood Glucose Level

Day/Date: Tuesday, January 23

Time/ meal	Diabetes medicines		Food		Carb count (choices/ grams)	Before lunch (noon)	Blood glucose results		
	Type	Amount	Type	Amount			1 hour (1 p.m.)	2 hours (2 p.m.)	3 hours (3 p.m.)
12:00 noon	Humalog	4 units	Pizza with extra cheese, pepperoni, and onions (regular crust)	3 medium slices	6/92 g	117	178	192	234
			Garden salad with Light Italian dressing	1 1/2 cups 2 T	0/5 g 0/2 g				
			Total		6/99 g				

What is important about protein and diabetes?

The current ADA nutrition recommendations suggest that people with diabetes get 10–20% of their daily calories from protein. However, a typical American consumes more than that. You can get the protein you need from either animal sources, such as poultry, dairy foods, and red meat, or from vegetable sources, such as soy, legumes, and grains.

Diabetic kidney disease is diagnosed when a protein (albumin) appears in the urine in the range of 3–300 milligrams per 24 hours. If you have this condition, you may need to consider eating less protein. Several small studies of people with diabetic kidney disease have shown that eating 0.3 grams of protein per pound of body weight per day slowed the progression of kidney disease. At this point, people with diabetic kidney disease are told to follow the adult Recommended Dietary Allowance (RDA) of 0.4 grams per kilogram of body weight, or about 10% of their daily calories. Two other therapies that help with the early stages of diabetic kidney disease are good blood pressure control and the use of medications called ACE inhibitors.

The ADA suggests that your health care provider measure your kidney function each year because the best way to prevent the progression of kidney disease is early detection and management. This is a simple urine test that can provide important information about how your kidneys are working.

How much protein should you eat?

Whether you follow the ADA guideline of 10–20% of calories or the U.S. Government recommended daily amount (RDA) for protein, which is slightly lower, you will probably need to trim down your portions of protein. The RDA for the average male is about 60–65 grams of protein and for the average female about 50–55 grams of protein. If we translate this into servings of protein, that's 2 to 3 (3-ounce) servings of cooked meat or meat substitutes per day. If you have evidence of kidney disease, make an effort to eat no more than this amount of protein. And there is some evidence that eating more vegetable protein foods such as soy products or legumes rather than animal protein foods may be less damaging to your kidneys.

Each ounce of protein food contains about 7 grams of protein. So, a 2-ounce serving of protein has 14 grams of protein and 3 ounces has 21 grams. The serving size of protein for your meal plan is usually 2–3 ounces of cooked protein. That is a piece of meat about the size of the palm of your hand. While an ounce of meat has 7 grams of protein, the differences in choices of meat decide the amount of fat in the serving (Table 6-5). The more fat, the more calories you get, too.

What is important about fat and diabetes?

When you have diabetes, you have an increased risk of developing heart disease. In fact, people with type 2 diabetes have 2–4 times greater risk of developing heart disease than people without diabetes. One problem is that many people with diabetes, particularly people with type 2 (insulin resistant) diabetes, have abnormal blood fat levels.

TABLE 6-5 The Differences in Meat Servings		
Type of meat (3 oz cooked)	Fat (g)	Calories
Very lean meats (white meat chicken, flounder)	0–1	105
Lean meat (tenderloin, dark meat chicken)	9	165
Medium-fat meats (ground beef, pork chops)	15	225
High-fat meats (country pork ribs, regular cheese)	24	300

See page 84 to learn some rules of thumb for converting raw weight to cooked weight for protein foods.

Usually, people with type 2 diabetes and people with type 1 diabetes who have lots of weight around their middle have an elevated triglyceride level and a low HDL (good) cholesterol level. In addition, people with type 2 diabetes have a high amount of the small, dense LDL (bad) cholesterol. This type of LDL may increase the appearance of heart disease even if the total LDL level is not that high, which is usually the case.

The risk of heart disease is the reason for one of the strongest diabetes nutrition recommendations: Eat less saturated fat. There are some quick ways to eat less saturated fat, total fat, and cholesterol. Choose lean, reduced-fat, low-fat, or fat-free foods. (Watch the carb content of these foods.) Prepare foods in low-fat ways, and eat small portions. Today there are many leaner cuts of meat, skinless chicken and turkey parts, reduced-fat cheeses, fat-free milk, and other lower-fat dairy foods to make your job of reducing saturated fat and cholesterol easier.

To determine how much fat and what types of fat to eat, you need to know whether your blood fat levels are normal (Table 6-6). The ADA recommends that adults with diabetes have their blood fats checked every year. If your levels fall into a lower risk category, you can have the test every two years. If your levels are abnormal, ask your health care professional to check them more often to see how you're progressing with treatment.

If you are at a healthy weight and have normal blood fat levels, you can eat 30% of your calories from fat, but saturated fat (butter, hard margarine, cream, bacon) should not account for more than 10% of your total calories. You want to keep polyunsaturated fats (mayonnaise; corn, soybean, or safflower oils) at or below 10% of your calories, too. Monounsaturated fats (canola, olive, or peanut oils; nuts; peanut butter; avocados) can be in the range of 10–15% of calories. Try to eat no more than 300 mg of cholesterol per day. If you want to lose weight, try reducing the calories from fat below 30%. If you have high triglycerides,

TABLE 6-6 Blood-Fat Goals with Diabetes*	
Total cholesterol	**<200 mg/dL**
LDL ("bad" cholesterol)	<100 mg/dl
HDL ("good" cholesterol)	>35 mg/dl
Triglycerides	<200 mg/dl

* Note the ADA recommendations for people with diabetes are slightly different from those for the general population without heart disease.

then lower your carbohydrate intake to about 40% of calories and increase your total fat calories to about 40% with monounsaturated fats contributing about 20% of those calories. **Don't let all these percentages confuse you, read on. And ask your dietitian for help.**

How much fat should you eat?

You do not need to eat a specific number of fat servings each day. Table 6-7 shows how many grams of fat to eat if you want 20, 30, or 40% of your calories from fat for various calorie levels.

TABLE 6-7 How Much Fat to Eat						
	Calorie level					
Total	**About 1200**	**About 1400**	**About 1600**	**About 1800**	**About 2200**	**About 2800**
Fat grams (20%)	27	31	36	40	49	62
Fat grams (30%)	40	47	53	60	73	93
Fat grams (40%)	53	62	71	80	98	124

What can you learn from the grams of total fat?

Are you a little curious about how you can figure how much total fat and the types of fats you need? Here's an example using 1500 calories.

Total number of calories: 1500
Multiply calories by 30%:   1500
$$\times\ .30$$
450 calories from fat

Divide calories from fat by 9 (9 calories per gram of fat):

$$\frac{450}{9} = 50 \text{ grams of total fat}$$

Now you can also figure the number of grams of saturated and polyunsaturated fat to eat so you can stay under 10% for each.

Multiply calories by 10%:   1500
$$\times\ .10$$
150 calories from fat

Divide this number by 9 (9 calories per gram of fat):

$$\frac{150}{9} = 17 \text{ grams of}$$
saturated and
17 grams of poly-
unsaturated fat

You can figure the number of grams of monounsaturated fat to eat for 10–15% of your daily calories. You already know that 10% of 1500 calories is 17 grams of fat. But to find the number of grams of monounsaturated fat in 15% of the 1500 calories you would:

Multiply calories by 15%: 1500
                          $\times .15$
                          225 calories from fat

Divide this number by 9 (9 calories per gram of fat):

$$\frac{225}{9} = 25 \text{ grams of monounsaturated fat}$$

Should you limit trans fats?

Trans fats are man-made, and there is growing evidence that the trans fats in many processed foods raise your cholesterol and your health risks to the point of making it well worth your time to limit them. You'll find trans fats in processed foods such as cookies, cake, chips, crackers, margarine, and microwave popcorn. Trans fats are not yet listed on the food label, but if you read the list of ingredients, and you see "partially hydrogenated vegetable oil" or "vegetable shortening," you've probably found the trans fats. Trans fats help foods hold their shape, which keeps stick margarine solid and store-bought cookies soft. It is a little ironic that you choose to eat margarine to avoid the saturated fat in butter, but the trans fats (hydrogenated fats) in the margarine raise the risk to your heart—perhaps even more. Look for margarine without trans fats, such as Promise or Benecol; there are some on the market. You can go for the soft spread, or make your own unsaturated spread by mixing one stick of butter with one cup of canola oil in a blender. Check your cookbooks for a recipe.

Do fat replacers contain carbohydrate?

The push to eat less fat has given rise to a flurry of reduced-fat, low-fat, and fat-free foods. When fat is removed from food to lower the fat content and calories, food manufacturers have to put something into the products to make them continue to taste good. Using ingredients that are called "fat replacers," manufacturers can make reduced-fat, low-fat, and fat-free foods, such as ice cream, sour cream, cream cheese, salad dressing, potato chips, and margarine. Fat replacers are ingredients that are made from carbohydrate, protein, or fat. An example of a carbohydrate-based fat replacer is maltodextrin, modified food starch. An example of a protein-based fat replacer is Simplesse; and an example of a fat-based fat replacer is olestra.

The majority of fat replacers in use today are made of carbohydrate. When the fat is taken out and these fat replacers are put in, the calories are usually, but not always, lower. But the carbohydrate content usually is higher.

For people with diabetes, especially those using carb counting, these extra grams of carbohydrate affect your meal plan. Ask your dietitian for help fitting these foods in. Read the Nutrition Facts labels on reduced-fat, low-fat, and fat-free foods to determine how to fit them into your meal plan. Then taste them. You may find a few lower-fat foods that you enjoy and want to use regularly. If you don't like the taste, there are other ways to lower the fat content of your meals.

7

The Size of Your Servings Is the Key to Success

You can eat only "healthy foods" and still gain weight. Healthy foods—such as whole-grain breads and cereals, fruits, and beans—do have calories in them, so it is possible to eat too much of them. Bottom line: It's not just a matter of what you eat, it's clearly also a matter of how much.

Surprisingly, the extra carbohydrate from servings that are *just a bit* too large can add up quickly. Perhaps you regularly eat an extra 1/2 cup of pasta or potatoes at dinner or a large apple rather than a small apple at lunch. And, it's not just the carbohydrate. It might be an extra ounce or two of meat (protein and fat) at dinner and an extra tablespoon of regular salad dressing (fat) at lunch. It is easy to rationalize that these extras could not be enough to prevent you from achieving blood glucose control or your other diabetes goals. After all you're not eating a candy bar or slice of cheesecake! That is true, but extra servings on a daily basis can mean the difference between hitting your blood glucose targets—or losing weight—and not.

Our Super-sized Society

In this society, it is a huge challenge to eat only the size portions we really need, with ever-larger dinner plates, super-sized fast food meals, and all-you-can-eat buffet restaurants.

For example, in a fast food restaurant, the difference in calories between a "value meal" and a "Super-sized value meal" is 600 calories! We've lost sight of reasonable portions. This is especially true for you if you frequently go to restaurants where common serving sizes are a 10-ounce steak, two cups of pasta, a three-egg omelet, or jumbo order of French fries. Clearly, these typical restaurant portions don't follow the serving sizes that we see on food Nutrition Facts labels or the servings suggested in this book. Unfortunately, these super-sized servings are leading to an obese population and an epidemic of type 2 diabetes.

What Size Serving?

It is likely that you already have all the tools you need to pinpoint the size of your servings. Do you have measuring spoons and measuring cups for liquids and solids? Most every household has these valuable kitchen utensils, but they're hidden away. Find them a new home—up front on the shelf nearest to the dishes that you use. You will be working with these tools at every meal for awhile. Table 7-1 can help you get comfortable with the weights and measures you'll be seeing often.

Here's what you need:

Measuring spoons. A set of measuring spoons with 1/2 teaspoon, 1 teaspoon, 1/2 tablespoon, and 1 tablespoon. When you use these measuring spoons, you'll see that there are 3 teaspoons in 1 tablespoon. Don't rely on your teaspoon and tablespoons from your silverware. They vary in size based on style and won't give you exact measurements.

Measuring cup—liquids. A 1-cup measuring cup with lines showing 1/4, 1/3, 1/2, 2/3, and 3/4 cup measures, too. A liquid measuring cup should be clear (glass or plastic) so you can see through it. To measure liquids correctly, set the cup down and bend down at eye level to make sure the liquid reaches the proper line.

Measuring cup—solids. A set of 1/4 cup, 1/2 cup, 3/4 cup, and 1 cup measuring cups. Choose the correct size for your serving, for example of cereal or rice, and fill it to the top. Level it with the flat edge of a knife. For instance, if you need 1/2 cup of uncooked hot cereal, measure it in a 1/2-cup measure and level it off with a flat knife to eliminate any excess.

Food Scale. Get at least an inexpensive ($5–10) food scale, particularly for measuring foods that don't have food labels, such as fresh fruit or bagels. You measure these foods in ounces—bagels, dinner rolls, baked potatoes, snack foods, cereals, baked goods, meats, fish, and cheese.

Upscale Food Scales. More expensive scales are available, but they are not necessary. You can spend a low of $25 to a high of $190. On the low end, the food scale measures ounces, pounds, grams, and kilograms. On the high end are digital scales that give you an exact measure rather than making you read between the lines. And there are scales that actually give you the gram weight of the food and the grams of carbohydrate in that amount of the food for about 400 common foods, such as the one made by Soehnle. The price is between $150–200.

TABLE 7-1 Common Household Measurements
3 teaspoons (tsp) = 1 tablespoon (Tbsp)
4 Tbsp = 1/4 cup = 2 fluid ounces
8 Tbsp = 1/2 cup = 4 fluid ounces
16 Tbsp = 1 cup = 8 fluid ounces
1 cup = 1/2 pint
2 cups = 1 pint
1 ounce = 30 grams (dry)

Eyes. Don't underestimate a well-trained and honest set of eyes. Your eyes are an invaluable measuring tool because you always have them with you.

The Nutrition Facts on the Food Label. The Nutrition Facts label on most packaged foods today is one of your best tools because it must list the serving size. Best yet, it's free and widely available. The serving sizes on food labels today, unlike those before 1994, are regulated by the FDA. These are the serving sizes that food manufacturers must use to comply with the food-labeling law. For us consumers, this is good news. All the packaged food manufacturers are using the same sizes of servings. This means that one serving of dry cereal is 30 grams or about 1 ounce for all dry cereals on the market. (Take care not to confuse the weight in grams of the serving with the grams of carbohydrate in the serving. Those are two different numbers.) Another helpful addition to the Nutrition Facts is the serving size in "common household terms," such as 7 crackers or 2/3 cup. That makes serving sizes easier to understand.

All the nutrition information on the Nutrition Facts label is based on one serving. Use the serving sizes to help you learn what reasonable portions are. If you usually eat a larger quantity of that food, perhaps your portions are too large or the portion you may be counting as one serving is actually two or three. It is important to say here that the food label serving size is not necessarily the same as a serving for carb counting or a serving on the Exchange Lists. For these meal-planning approaches, one serving (or choice) has 15 grams of carbohydrate. If you use the "carbohydrate choice" system, you can use the grams of carbohydrate on the Nutrition Facts label to figure how much food to eat to match the number of carbohydrate choices you want.

For example, look at the Nutrition Facts panel for a cold cereal on page 80. It says a 1-ounce (or 1 cup) serving is 37 grams of carbohydrate. When you divide 37 by 15, you see that this serving is 2 carbohydrate choices with 7 grams of carbohydrate left over. If you look at the chart on page 23, you will see that 7 grams of carbohydrate is 1/2 carbohydrate choice. So, a serving of one cup of this cereal is 2 1/2 carbohydrate choices. If you are counting carbohydrate by grams, you just check the serving size and grams of total carbohydrate on the label and make sure your serving size is the same. Or you adjust your carb count for the size of the serving you eat.

The Nutrition Facts panel is an excellent resource for learning about the carbohydrate content of foods. Nearly all Nutrition Facts labels provide the grams of Total Carbohydrate (chapter 8).

Nutrition Facts

Serving Size 1 cup (56g)
Servings Per Container about 8

Amount Per Serving	Cereal alone	with 1/2 cup skim milk
Calories	120	160
Calories from Fat	10	10
	% Daily Value**	
Total Fat 1g*	**2%**	**3%**
Saturated Fat 0g	**0%**	**0%**
Polyunsaturated Fat 0.5g		
Monounsaturated Fat 0g		
Cholesterol 0mg	**0%**	**1%**
Sodium 150mg	**16%**	**19%**
Potassium 80mg	**6%**	**12%**
Total Carbohydrate 37g	**16%**	**18%**
Dietary Fiber 2g	**30%**	**30%**
Sugars 9g		
Other Carbohydrate 26g		
Protein 3g		

When to Weigh and Measure

It is particularly important to weigh and measure your foods as you begin to count carbohydrates. If you weigh and measure all your foods and beverages for a couple of weeks, you will learn a lot about the correct serving size and maybe some surprising facts about your usual serving size. Don't worry, you do not have to weigh and measure foods every day for years to come! That's not practical or realistic, especially when you eat away from home. Keep in mind, however, that the more often you practice weighing and measuring foods and beverages at home, the easier it is to estimate correct servings when you eat away from home.

Always weigh or measure new foods. Occasionally weigh or measure foods and beverages you regularly eat to check that your eyes are still seeing correct serving sizes—those portions can slowly grow over time. Another time to go back to weighing and measuring foods is when you see your blood glucose levels or your weight start to climb. Perhaps one reason these numbers are on the rise is that your portions have grown. The bottom line for mastering serving sizes is honesty. If you are honest with yourself, your servings will be on the money more times than not.

Tips and Tricks

To help you see servings, here are some "handy" guidelines.

Thumb tip = 1 tsp	Example: 1 tsp mayonnaise, salad dressing, or margarine
Thumb = 1 oz	Example: 1 oz cheese or meat
Palm = 3 oz	Example: 3 oz cooked meat (boneless)
Tight Fist = 1/2 cup	Example: 1 serving noodles or rice, 1 serving canned fruit
Loose fist = 1 cup	Example: 1 cup vegetables
Handful = 1 cup	Example: 2 servings pasta, 2 servings cooked vegetable
2 bars of hotel soap	2 small cookies
4 oz wine	a cupcake wrapper

These guidelines hold true for most women's hands, but some men's hands are much larger. Check it out for yourself!

At home, always serve meals in the same size plates, glasses, and bowls. This technique helps you judge correct portions, and you don't have to use the measuring tools so often. For instance, use the same glass each time you drink milk. Measure your serving into a measuring cup once or twice. Pour it into the glass. See where your serving comes to in the glass. You can mark it if you want with an indelible marker or piece of masking tape. Every now and then, measure your serving in a measuring cup to check your accuracy. You need to see how much room 1 cup of pasta takes on a dinner plate, 1/2 cup of hot oatmeal in a bowl, and so on. Keep these "pictures" in your mind.

Once you feel confident that you can eyeball serving sizes correctly and honestly, you don't have to weigh and measure everything. It's wise to do so from time to time, perhaps once a week on Monday, just to make sure your eyes don't lose the picture over time. You can quiz yourself occasionally. Pour the amount of dry cereal, pasta, or rice you usually eat into the container you eat it in. Then measure the quantity you poured. Is the serving size correct? If not, you can readjust your eyeballs by using the measuring tools for a week or two.

If you serve family style meals—that means filling large serving bowls and putting them on the table for everyone to help themselves—think about serving in the kitchen. This style of serving food promotes overeating. Seconds are that much closer to your fork and lips. Dish up servings on plates in the kitchen. If people want seconds, they have to walk for them.

When you purchase fresh produce (fruits and vegetables) take advantage of the food scales that hang in the market produce area. Weigh individual pieces of fruit. Focus on what a 4-ounce banana, 6 1/2-ounce orange, or 3 1/2-ounce kiwi really looks like. These all represent 1 carbohydrate choice or 15 grams of carbohydrate. Think about your eating habits. Do you reach for the largest apple or banana and count it as 1 serving or 15 grams of carbohydrate, but it's really 1 1/2 carb servings or 22 grams of carbohydrate or even 2 carb choices and 30 grams of carbohydrate? Measure pieces of fruit on the food scale in the produce area on several shopping trips. This will help cement a visual picture in your mind of the correct serving of fruit. Then buy the pieces of food that fit your needs on each shopping trip. To keep yourself in check, weigh your produce on occasion to make sure your visual picture is still sharp. Note that the weights listed for one serving of fresh fruits in carb counting food lists include the skin, core, seeds, and rind.

It's easy to go overboard on servings of meat, poultry, and cheese because one more ounce does not look like that much more. However, it adds another 35–100 calories, depending on the fat content, for each extra ounce. Try this. When you buy a package of cheese, cold cuts, or anything you buy by the ounce, glance at the ounces on the label. Then visualize what 1, 2, or 3 ounces looks like. If you buy cheese or cold cuts sliced to order, think about how many meals you will make from that quantity. Let that be your guide to how many ounces you buy. If you make a smoked turkey and Swiss cheese sandwich for lunch with 2 ounces of turkey and 1 ounce of cheese, how many sandwiches are you going to make until the next time you shop? Buy the amount you need, not just any amount. Another benefit is that you waste less food.

When you purchase a piece of meat, such as pork roast, leg of lamb, or chicken breasts, estimate the amount of raw meat you need to buy. Think about how many people you are feeding, what quantity you will lose in cooking (see the rule of thumb on page 84) and how much you want for leftovers. That's your number. Write it by the item on your shopping list or do your calculations at the meat counter.

Meet Rita Rita has been overweight for a number of years now. She is 52 and about a year ago found out that she has type 2 diabetes. Her nurse practitioner put her on a diabetes medication that

RAW TO COOKED: RULES OF THUMB

Raw meat with no bone: 4 oz raw to get 3 oz cooked.

Raw meat with bone: 5 oz raw to get 3 oz cooked.

Raw poultry with skin: 4 1/4–4 1/2 oz to get 3 oz cooked. The extra 1/4 to 1/2 oz accounts for the skin. (Remove the skin before or after cooking.)

Here is an example for a whole chicken: Each family member needs about 3 oz cooked chicken. There are 5 family members. The chicken has bones and skin, so you need to figure about 5 1/2 oz per person. So, 5 × 5 1/2 = 28 oz or about 1 3/4 pounds. If you want enough for two meals, you need about 3 1/2 pounds. Do not forget a few ounces for the organs stuffed in the cavity. So, you need about a 4-pound chicken.

initially helped lower her blood glucose levels, but eventually, she put on another 12 pounds rather than losing weight. Every time Rita came to see the nurse practitioner, she advised Rita to eat less and exercise more. Each time Rita returned, the scale would show a few more pounds— she was up to 183 pounds. That was the most she had ever weighed and was way too much on her 5'4" frame. She was frustrated and didn't feel like she could get her diabetes in control. The nurse practitioner suggested she see a dietitian. When she made the appointment, the receptionist gave her forms on which to keep food records for the two weeks before she came to see the dietitian. She was also encouraged to bring her meter and blood glucose monitoring records for her visit.

Rita came to see the dietitian with all her records in hand. After they got acquainted, the dietitian reviewed Rita's food records with her. The dietitian noted that Rita just wrote down the types of foods she ate, but not the amounts. It was clear that Rita was, generally speaking, choosing healthy foods to eat. When the dietitian asked Rita if she weighed or measured her foods, Rita said she didn't think it was necessary if she was eating healthy foods and watching her fat intake. The dietitian pointed out that because Rita has to count her calories to lose some weight, she would do better if she weighed and measured her foods as often as possible, especially when she eats at home.

The dietitian began to teach Rita basic carb counting and encouraged her to choose 3 servings of carbohydrate at breakfast, 4 at lunch, and 5 at dinner. The dietitian showed Rita some food models of the serving sizes she should eat. Rita was amazed at how small the portions looked. The dietitian asked Rita what measuring tools she had at home. Rita said she has measuring cups and spoons but doesn't have a food scale. The dietitian encouraged Rita to use her tools, particularly to measure foods like pasta, dry cereal, rice, potatoes, and milk. Since Rita has been going a bit wild on fresh fruit, the dietitian discussed reasonable servings of these foods. The dietitian encouraged Rita to look for smaller pieces of fruit.

Rita left the dietitian's office both pleased and disappointed. She was pleased that they identified her servings as a problem area. She believes that if she watches her portions more carefully, she will lose weight and get her blood glucose levels into better control. But she was disappointed because she knows she cannot eat as much as she has been eating.

Rita went back to see the dietitian in 4 weeks. She brought along her Carbohydrate Counts and Blood Glucose Results Record that the dietitian asked her to keep. This time she had filled in the amounts of the foods she ate. She was pleased because her weight was down 1 1/2 pounds. No longer on the rise! And her blood glucose results had inched down as well. She says that since she has been weighing and measuring her foods, she laughs as she realizes how much she was eating. She believes she can continue to lose weight if she continues to be honest about how much she eats. The dietitian suggested that Rita add some physical activity to her schedule. She noted that even a small amount of activity each day would help burn calories and blood glucose. Rita is going to try to do more gardening this summer and to take a 15-minute walk 2–3 evenings a week.

Rita came back for a third visit two months later with her records in hand. She was scheduled to see both her nurse practitioner and dietitian. Sure enough, she got on the scale, and it showed a weight loss of 3 pounds over two months. Her weight was dropping into the 170s. Her blood glucose levels had inched down some more. The best news was that her HbA_{1c} had inched down too, from 9.2% to 8.4%. Both of her clinicians said that was terrific. They complimented her on her hard work taking care of her diabetes. She and the dietitian talked about strategies for controlling serving sizes at restaurants because Rita mentioned that she had been staying away from them. They also talked about some reduced-fat and low-sugar products that might be helpful to Rita.

8

The Food Label Has the Facts

T oday supermarkets are nutrient data warehouses. The Nutrition Facts labels on most food packages is there because of the revolutionary changes in the food labeling law that went into effect in 1994. These laws were written and are enforced by the Food and Drug Administration (FDA) and U.S. Department of Agriculture (USDA). The Nutrition Facts label is one of the most complete and up-to-date sources for the nutrient content of the foods you choose to eat. And it's free! There's no charge for reading the fine print or for comparing the numbers on several different labels.

As a carb counter, you'll find that the listing for total carbohydrate in the Nutrition Facts is worth its weight in gold. It's helpful as you learn the carbohydrate content of the foods you eat and when you want to choose new foods.

What foods have a Nutrition Facts label?

Almost all packaged and processed foods have Nutrition Facts labels. There are a few exceptions—fresh fruits, vegetables, fresh meat, poultry, and fish. Carb counting resources (Appendix 1) can help you find the amount of carb in these foods.

What's on the Nutrition Facts label?

To get you better acquainted with the Nutrition Facts panel information, let's look at a label from a box of whole-grain dry cereal.

Nutrition Facts

Serving Size 1 cup (58g)

Servings Per Container about 8

Amount Per Serving	Multi-Bran Chex	with 1/2 cup skim milk
Calories	200	240
Calories from Fat	15	15
	% Daily Value**	
Total Fat 1.5g*	**2%**	**3%**
Saturated Fat 0g	**0%**	**0%**
Polyunsaturated Fat 0.5g		
Monounsaturated Fat 0g		
Cholesterol 0mg	**0%**	**1%**
Sodium 380mg	**16%**	**19%**
Potassium 220mg	**6%**	**12%**
Total Carbohydrate 49g	**16%**	**18%**
Dietary Fiber 8g	**30%**	**30%**
Sugars 12g		
Other Carbohydrate 29g		
Protein 4g		

Nutrition Facts

Nutrition Facts is the title of the list of information about the food. Manufacturers are required to use it and give all the nutrient information in the same format. This is the first time that the law has required manufacturers to use a standard, easy-to-read label. The information under the Nutrition Facts heading tells you the serving size, the number of servings in the container, calories, calories from fat, total fat, saturated fat, sodium, total carbohydrate, dietary fiber, sugars, protein, vitamins, and minerals for one serving of the food.

Serving Size. All the nutrition information on the label is based on one serving, **not the whole package** or container. The 1994 law created several improvements to make this information more valuable:

1. Serving sizes are uniform because the FDA established servings for 139 categories of foods, and manufacturers must use those servings.
2. So-called "reference amounts" are based on the amount of the food that people usually eat.
3. Serving size must be listed in both common household (for example: 4 crackers or 3/4 cup of pasta noodles) as well as metric measures (for example: 28 grams).

Servings Per Container. This is the number of servings in the container. Be sure to check this number before you eat everything in the box.

Calories. This is the number of calories in one serving, listed in bold print.

Calories from Fat. Manufacturers get this number from multiplying the number of grams of fat by 9, because there are 9 calories in 1 gram of fat.

Total Fat. The total grams of fat in the serving are listed in bold print.

Saturated Fat. The grams of saturated fat are listed under total fat, indented and not in bold print. Saturated fat is part of the total fat. The saturated fat is the only type of fat that must be listed on the label.

Polyunsaturated Fat and Monounsaturated Fat. These are listed under total fat, indented and not in bold print. These types of fat are listed voluntarily or if the manufacturer makes a nutrition claim about them.

Cholesterol. The milligrams of cholesterol are listed per serving in bold print.

Sodium. The milligrams of sodium are listed per serving in bold print.

Total Carbohydrate. All the grams of carbohydrate in one serving are listed in bold print. This number includes dietary fiber, sugars, and other sources of carbohydrate.

Dietary Fiber. The grams of dietary fiber per serving are listed under Total Carbohydrate and indented because fiber is part of the carbohydrate.

There are different types of fiber in foods, and all are considered carbohydrate. However, for the most part, they can't be digested, so they can't be turned into glucose for energy or raise blood sugar levels. There are two main types of dietary fiber—insoluble and soluble. Some food manufacturers do list the amount of soluble or insoluble fiber in a product if they have something to brag about or if they have to because they have made a nutrition claim about the product's fiber content.

If there are more than 5 grams of fiber in the serving that you eat, you should subtract the number of grams of fiber from the grams of total carbohydrate. Use that number for the carb count in the food. The carb from fiber will not raise your blood glucose. See page 154.

FIBER CLAIMS ON THE FOOD LABEL	
Fiber Term	**Means**
High or excellent source	5 grams or more of fiber per serving
Good source	2.5 to 4.9 grams per serving
More, enriched, or added	at least 2.5 grams per serving

Sugars. The grams of sugars per serving are listed under total carbohydrate and indented because sugars are part of the carbohydrate in the food. Many people with diabetes zero right in on the sugars. There is no need to do this! When you read the Nutrition Facts, look at the grams of total carbohydrate **only.** You don't need to single out the grams of sugars. When you count the carbohydrates, you have already counted the sugars.

Protein. The grams of protein per serving are in bold print.

Vitamins and Minerals. There are Recommended Daily Intake (RDI) levels for certain vitamins and minerals. The food label must list the percentage of the RDI for two vitamins—A and C—and two minerals—calcium and iron. Other vitamins and minerals are listed if the manufacturer makes claims about them. They can also be listed voluntarily. For example, if a food is fortified with folic acid, the Nutrition Facts must state the amount of folic acid per serving.

The Nutrition Facts label does not make it easy to interpret the amount of a vitamin or mineral in foods. Most people don't know the RDI amounts for vitamins and minerals. Without these numbers in hand, it is difficult to make any sense out of the information on the label. Table 8-1 gives the RDIs and may help you understand these percentages and make sense of claims on the label. For example, if you look at the label of fat-free milk, you see that a serving has 30% of the RDI for calcium. If you know that the RDI for calcium is 1000 mg, then you can multiply 1000 by .30, to discover that the milk has about 300 mg per 8-oz serving.

Here's another tip. If a manufacturer uses the terms "excellent source of, rich in, or high in," the product must contain at least 20% of the RDI for the vitamin or mineral named. If a manufacturer uses the terms "good source of, contains, or provides," the product must contain between 10–19% of the RDI for that vitamin or mineral. Table 8-1 also provides the amounts of the vitamins and minerals that

TABLE 8-1 The Daily Values and Label Claims for Vitamins and Minerals

Nutrient	Daily value	Excellent source of, rich in, high (20% or greater)	Good source of, contains, provides (10% to 19%)
Potassium	3500 mg	700 mg	350–665 mg
Dietary fiber	25/2000 cal	5 g	2.5–5 g
Vitamin A	5000 IU	1000 IU	500–950 IU
Vitamin C	90 mg (75 mg)	12 mg	6–11 mg
Calcium*	1000 mg	200 mg	100–190 mg
Iron	18 mg	3.6 mg	1.8–3.4 mg
Vitamin D	400 IU	80 IU	40–76 IU
Vitamin E	15 IU (12 IU)	6 IU	3–5.7 IU
Thiamin	1.5 mg	0.3 mg	0.15–0.29 mg
Riboflavin	1.7 mg	0.34 mg	0.17–0.32 mg
Niacin	20 mg	4 mg	2–3.8 mg
Vitamin B6	2 mg	0.4 mg	0.2–0.38 mg
Folate	400 mcg	80 mcg	40–76 mcg
Vitamin B12	6.0 mcg	1.2 mcg	0.6–1.14 mcg
Biotin	0.3 mg	0.06 mg	0.03–0.057 mg
Pantothenic acid	10 mg	2 mg	1–1.9 mg
Phosphorus	1000 mg	200 mg	100–190 mg
Iodine	150 mcg	30 mcg	15–29 mg
Magnesium	400 mg	80 mg	40–76 mg
Zinc	15 mg	3 mg	1.5–2.9 mg
Copper	2.0 mg	0.4 mg	0.2–0.38 mg

*Note:
Calcium: Adults over 51 have a calcium goal of 1200 mg/day.

must be present in a food before "excellent source of" or "good source of" claims can be made.

Other Nutrition Claims

Food manufacturers can make other claims on the food label, such as that the food is calorie free or sugar free. But what do these claims mean? There are guidelines for these claims set up by the food labeling laws. For an explanation of what they mean, see Table 8-2.

More about Sugars

It is important to understand that the word "sugars" on the Nutrition Facts panel can only, by FDA definition, be from one-unit sugars—glucose, fructose, galactose—or two-unit sugars—lactose, sucrose, or maltose. These sugars can be:

- Natural sugars, such as the lactose in milk or the sucrose in fruit.

Table 8-2. Nutrition Claims on the Food Label	
Nutrition claim	Means
Calorie free	Less than 5 calories per serving
Fat free	Less than 0.5 g fat per serving
Sugar free	Less than 0.5 g sugars per serving
Reduced calorie	At least 25% fewer calories than regular food
Reduced fat	At least 25% less fat than regular food
Reduced sugars	At least 25% less sugar than regular food
No added sugar, without added sugar, no sugar added	Permitted if no amount of sugars or ingredient that substitutes for sugar is used, contains no fruit juice concentrate or jelly, and the label says the food is not low calorie

■ Added sugars, such as corn sweeteners, high-fructose corn syrup, fruit juice, molasses, and brown sugar.

Because sugars in foods are from both natural and added sources, there is no way to tell by looking at the grams of sugars on the Nutrition Facts what the sources are. Check for sources of added sugars on the ingredient list. If the added sugars start to stack up, it tells you something about how nutritious—or not—the food is. Perhaps it's best left on the shelf.

Sugar Alcohols: Another Carbohydrate?

Yes, sugar alcohols are considered a source of carbohydrate. They are a group of carbohydrates that have a lower calorie count than other carbohydrates. Another name for this category of sweeteners is polyols. Sugar alcohols are neither sugars nor alcohol. Sugar alcohols provide, on average, 2 calories per gram, whereas other carbohydrates are 4 calories per gram. They are used by food manufacturers to replace sugars or fat and create foods that are lower in calories, sugar, or fat. Often times they are used to replace the bulk or volume that sugar gives to products. While you may want to reduce calories and choose lots of foods with sugar alcohols in them, be aware that sugar alcohols have a laxative side-effect on some people.

Polyols are most commonly used in candies, cookies, chewing gum, drinks, puddings, and sugar-free cough drops and breath mints. The names of polyols are easily recognized in the ingredients because most of them end in "ol," such as lactitol, mannitol, sorbitol, and xylitol. Isomalt and hydrogenated starch hydrolysates are two polyols that don't end in "ol." If a manufacturer makes a nutrition claim that the food is sugar free or has no added sugar, and it contains a sugar alcohol, then they must put the grams of sugar alcohols on the Nutrition Facts under total carbohydrate. See the food label for sugar-free gum.

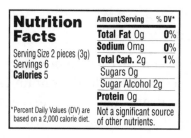

Nutrition Facts	Amount/Serving	% DV*
	Total Fat 0g	**0%**
Serving Size 2 pieces (3g)	**Sodium** 0mg	**0%**
Servings 6	**Total Carb.** 2g	**1%**
Calories 5	Sugars 0g	
	Sugar Alcohol 2g	
	Protein 0g	
*Percent Daily Values (DV) are based on a 2,000 calorie diet.	Not a significant source of other nutrients.	

How do you fit in foods with polyols?

If you choose to use foods with polyols, you need to count them into your meal plan.

Here are guidelines:

1. If all the total carbohydrate in the food comes from sugar alcohols and there are less than 10 grams in a serving, count the food as a free food. Remember that a free food has up to 20 calories and 5 grams of carbohydrate per serving. Limit free foods to 3 or fewer servings per day or the calories and carbohydrate will add up and keep you from meeting your diabetes goals.

2. If all the carbohydrate in the food comes from sugar alcohols and the grams of polyols are greater than 10 (look at the grams of total carbohydrate and grams of sugar alcohols), then subtract one-half of the grams of sugar alcohols from the total carbohydrate and count the remaining grams of carbohydrate.

3. If there are several sources of carbohydrate, which includes sugar alcohols (look at the grams of total carbohydrate and grams of sugar alcohols), then subtract one-half of the grams of sugar alcohols from the total carbohydrate and count the remaining grams of carbohydrate.

Low-Calorie Sweeteners: Another Carbohydrate?

No. Low-calorie sweeteners, more precisely called nonnutritive sweeteners because they don't contain calories, are not a source of carbohydrate. There are currently four nonnutritive sweeteners approved for use by the FDA—acesulfame-potassium, aspartame, saccharin, and sucralose. These sweeteners are in a multitude of foods and beverages on the supermarket shelves today, from packets to diet soda, hot cocoa, yogurt, syrup, and many others. Because low-calorie sweeteners don't contain any carbohydrate, they don't have to be accounted for on the Nutrition Facts label. However, because they are an ingredient in the foods, they must be listed in the ingredients list.

Fitting in Foods with Low-Calorie Sweeteners

If you choose to use foods with low-calorie sweeteners, you need to know how much carbohydrate they contain from other ingredients. Products sweetened with no-calorie sweeteners can be divided into three categories.

Here are some guidelines for using them:

1. Tabletop sweeteners come in packets or granular form of a low-calorie sweetener that usually has about 2 calories for the equivalent sweetness of 2 teaspoons of sugar. The calories are not from the low-calorie sweetener but from the dextrose or maltodextrin that is used to give bulk or volume to the product. These are negligible calories and are considered free foods unless you consume large amounts.
2. Foods with low-calorie sweeteners that contain few calories, such as diet soda, diet gelatin, chewing gum, fruit drinks, and powdered drink mix. As long as the Nutrition Facts tell you that a serving is less than 5 grams of carbohydrate, consider this a free food and consume these products in reasonable amounts.

3. Foods sweetened with low-calorie sweeteners, such as hot cocoa mix, yogurt with fruit, maple syrup, baked goods, frozen desserts, canned fruit, and fruit drink, may contain other ingredients that contribute carbohydrate, nutrients, and calories. If the Nutrition Facts tell you that a serving has more than 5 grams of carbohydrate, you need to fit these foods into your meal plan the same as you fit in any other food with carbohydrate. See Table 8-3 for examples of food label information for different versions of ice cream—regular, light, low fat, fat free, and fat free/no sugar added. Every type of ice cream has carb that you need to count in your meal plan.

Try Your Hand at Using Food Labels

It will be important for you to be able to use the Nutrition Facts label to do carb counting. Here are a few practice experiences.

TABLE 8-3 Food Labels for Ice Cream (1/2 cup [4 oz] serving)				
	Regular*	Light/ low fat	Fat free/ no sugar added†	Fat Free
Calories	160	100	90	110
Total Fat	9	3	0	0
Saturated Fat	5	2	0	0
Cholesterol	50	20	0	0
Total Carbohydrate	17	15	19	24
Protein	2	3	3	3

* Not super premium high fat ice cream.
† Contains sugar alcohols/polyols.

1. I often eat cooked oat bran cereal for breakfast. The Nutrition Facts say one serving is 1/3 cup and 1 serving contains 19 grams of carbohydrate and 5 grams of fiber. I eat 2/3 cup as a serving. How many carbohydrate choices are in my serving and do I need to subtract the fiber content?

The serving size of 2/3 cup cooked oat bran contains 38 g carbohydrate (19 g + 19 g) and 10 g fiber (5 g + 5 g). You should subtract the grams of fiber because there are more than 5 grams. So 38 g carbohydrate – 10 g fiber = 28 g carb or about 2 carb choices. (Round up to 30 g carb or 2 carb choices.) If you add milk or raisins, or eat other sources of carbohydrate with this breakfast, you will need to add those carbs to your total.

2. For dinner you decide to eat the following foods. You read the total carbohydrate on the Nutrition Facts panel for the manicotti, salad dressing, and yogurt. You check the carb count books to get the carb counts for each food that doesn't have a Nutrition Facts label: the roll, salad, and strawberries. Write them down and add it all up.

Item	Carbohydrate (g)
Three-cheese manicotti frozen entrée	41
1 dinner roll	19
1 cup salad greens	–
2 Tbsp fat-free Catalina dressing	11
1 1/4 cup sliced strawberries	15
1/2 cup orange frozen yogurt	26
Total carbohydrate	112

If you use carbohydrate choices, how many choices would this meal add up to?

112 g carb ÷ 15 = 7.7 carb choices or servings, round up to 8
Answer: 8

   3. I often eat dry cereal for a quick breakfast. I mix
      three cereals together to get a bunch of fiber and the
      taste I enjoy. I also add 2 tablespoons of raisins.
      What's the total carbohydrate count for this
      breakfast?

Item	My cereal (g carb)	Nutrition Facts (g carb)
1/2 cup Wheaties	12	24 g in 1 cup
1/2 cup Shredded Wheat	23	47 g in 1 cup
1/3 cup low fat Granola	24	48 g in 2/3 cup
2 Tbsp raisins	15	15
1 cup fat-free milk	12	12
Total carb count	86	79

My servings of the three cereals are half of the serving sizes
listed on the Nutrition Facts panels. I remembered to add
the carb count for the raisins and milk, too.

How many carb choices is this breakfast?
86 ÷ 15 = 5 11/15 or round up to 6 carb choices
Answer: 6

Bonus question #1: Your cereal breakfast has fiber in it.
1.5 g + 2.5 g + 2 g + 1 g = 7 g fiber. What is the carb count
of this breakfast?

86 − 7 = 79 g carb

Bonus question #2: How many units of insulin would you
need to cover this breakfast if you took 1 unit for each 17
grams of carbohydrate?

112 ÷ 17 = 5 1/17; round down to 5
Answer: 5 units of insulin

9

Beyond Meat and Potatoes

E ating out at restaurants or bringing take-out food home is the American way of life these days. Most of us eat 3–4 meals away from home each week. Or we buy convenience or packaged foods from supermarkets to save us preparation and cooking time. Your eating style does not have to change because you want to use carb counting. In fact, when you get practiced at using carb counting, you may well enjoy going out to eat even more because you have tools to take the uncertainty out of what your meals will do to your blood sugar level.

Meet George
George ate quite a few packaged foods every day, such as frozen pizza, frozen waffles, and boxed macaroni and cheese. He was a very bright young man and always in a hurry. His work schedule had changed, so he was eating breakfast at the early hour of 6 a.m. and lunch was not until 11:30. Around 9 a.m., he was eating a cookie from the vending machine. It was called a Monster cookie, and he checked the total carbohydrate on the food label. It was 35 grams of total carbohydrate. When he checked his blood glucose before lunch or 2 hours after eating the cookie, it was in the 220–250 mg/dl range. This happened 3 days in a row. He didn't know why his blood sugar was running

high, so he called his dietitian. He had faxed her a copy of the label. She checked the serving size and it was 1 cookie. There were 2 cookies in the package, and he was eating them both. His morning snack contained 70 grams of carbohydrate. Then he realized that he had not been checking the serving size and the number of servings per package. These numbers are as important as the number of grams of carbohydrate. He and his dietitian discussed a plan for better control: to eat more breakfast to prevent low blood glucose mid-morning and eliminate the need for the cookie snack—or to find some healthier snacks.

Restaurant Foods: Eat In or Take Out

You can use this activity to get a clearer idea of your restaurant eating habits.

1. Which meals and snacks do you eat away from home, during the day, week, or month? Are you more likely to eat out during the day or the evening?
2. Why do you eat meals at a restaurant?

   - Convenience
   - Lack of time
   - To get a variety of foods
   - Not interested in cooking
   - Like to be served
   - Food tastes good

3. What type of foods do you eat at restaurants? In what quantities? Write down what you eat and try to estimate the size of the serving and the amount of carbohydrates in it. If you have information on your blood glucose levels after eating out, put those down, too. These records will provide clues about how well you are estimating the carbohydrate in your restaurant meals. Also write down the beverages you drink,

whether they are carbonated, fruit juices, alcoholic, or calorie free. Some of these beverages have carbohydrates and calories, and you may not realize how much you are consuming.

Now, do you have a better picture of your eating-out style? Your records provide the data you need to count the carb choices or grams of carbohydrate in the foods you eat away from home. Check the food lists in this book or in other books to help you count the carbs in your favorite restaurant meals, often-used convenience foods, or snacks from the vending machine at work. When you eat out, do you follow your meal plan or ignore it? Do you overeat in certain restaurants or at certain times of the day? What can you learn about yourself from your food records? You can usually get the menu from your favorite restaurants—even fast food places—and make a list of the dishes you order and figure the carb counts before you go there again. Add to your book of carb counts the restaurant foods that you frequently eat—pizza, burger and fries, Chinese food—by listing food/amount/carb.

Restaurant Eating: Tips and Skills

Eating the correct size serving is a challenge in restaurants. First, the portions are generally huge. It's up to you to figure out ways to eat only the servings you need. If you practice weighing and measuring your servings at home, your skills will be ready for the restaurant challenge. Your well-trained eyes help you estimate portions. The more you can visualize proper servings, the easier it is to follow your eating plan.

Here are a few tips for eating restaurant meals:

■ Be on the lookout for the words on the menu that mean large portions—large, giant, grande, supreme, extra large, jumbo, double, triple, double-decker, king-size, and super. Search for the words that mean small portions—junior, single, petite, kiddie, and regular. No surprise, these are harder to find.

- If you see a weight for a piece of meat on the menu, it's most likely the raw weight. For example, you might see a hamburger referred to as a "quarter pound" of meat or a filet weighing 6 ounces, or a slice of prime rib that weighs 10 ounces. Remember that these are average—not exact—weights. Apply the rule of thumb on page 84 to help you convert servings from raw weight to cooked weight. Also keep in mind that entrée portions of meat in sit-down restaurants are often enough for two people.

- Think about ordering a soup and salad, or appetizer and soup. That may be enough for you. Or see if you can order a half portion. This is particularly easy to do with pasta entrées. Ask whether your dining partner is willing to share. For example, in a steak house, one person orders the steak (which is enough for two) and the other person orders side orders of a baked potato, salad, or vegetable. Consider splitting two entrees that complement each other. For example, in an Italian restaurant, one person orders pasta topped with a tomato-based sauce and the other orders a chicken, veal, or fish dish. Split both dishes and you've each got a more balanced meal. Or you can all eat family style—share several dishes among several people. Just order fewer dishes than the number of mouths at the table.

- Know when enough is enough. Don't clean your plate. Take the extras home. It's a good idea not to wait until you're stuffed to figure out what the extras are. Ask for a take-home container when you order your meal. Divide the meal and put the half you don't really want to eat in the container before you start.

- You might want to go a step further than just eye-balling portions, especially if your blood glucose seems to be hard to control after your favorite restaurant meals. You could order one or two of your favorite items to take home. At home, carefully weigh and measure the portions. See if your eyeball measurements are accurate or if you greatly under- or over-estimated. The next time you order that food in your favorite restaurant, you will be able to adjust your medication more precisely to control your blood glucose levels. Or you may eat more carefully, so you get only the serving you need. (You might decide to eat a higher carbohydrate, protein, and fat meal either at home or in a restaurant. For those of you who adjust your insulin doses, see chapter 12.)

■ There are several resources to help you better estimate the nutrition in restaurant foods (Appendix 2).

■ See the Handy Hand Guides on pages 81. It is not practical to carry a food scale or measuring cups to a restaurant. These memory guides can help you guess-timate the size of your servings when you eat in restaurants, at a friend or relative's house, or even when you eat at home and feel you have mastered weighing and measuring your foods. Blood glucose checks before and after restaurant meals is the best tool to see if you are truly on target with the amount of carbohydrate in the meal.

Meet JB   JB ate all his lunches at the food court of the local mall during the workweek. He rotated his choices from the various ethnic cafes at the food court. The selections varied among Greek, Chinese, Japanese, Mexican, and Italian. He had the habit of ordering the same item from each of the places, and he selected each one on a specific day. He was concerned about his blood glucose levels, and he had learned by keeping a food and blood glucose record that with some meals he had great glucose levels after the meal and with others his levels were too high. He was trying to eat a certain range of carbohydrate grams. So his dietitian suggested that they do a "food lab" with his food choices. He bought one of each item that he usually ordered, and they measured the carb counts of each. His target for grams of carbohydrates at lunch was 60–75 grams. Typically, he orders:

Chinese: vegetable stir-fry with a bowl of fried rice

Mexican: 2 beef enchiladas (small)

Greek: a gyro sandwich with cucumber salad

Japanese: a plate of sushi with miso soup

Italian: 2 slices of deep-dish pizza with a small garden salad and Thousand Island dressing

He and his dietitian measured the servings with measuring cups and a food scale to figure the actual amount of carbs in each meal. JB thought all of them contained between 60–75 grams of carbohydrate.

Chinese. They measured the amount of fried rice in the bowl. It should have been 2 1/2 cups. The actual amount was 4 1/2 cups, which has 135 grams of carbohydrate. The stir-fry veggies were all non-starchy vegetables, like broccoli and bok choy, and there was 1 cup of them, or 10 grams of carb. This meal had 140 grams of carb, which was nearly twice as much as the 60–75 gram target range. When he checked his blood glucose level after the meal, it was 200 mg/dl. This showed that the larger amount of carbs raised his blood glucose higher than he wanted it to be 2 hours after the meal.

Mexican. His 2 beef enchiladas had 35 grams of carbohydrate—much less than his target level. When he checked his blood glucose level 2 hours later, it was 60 mg/dl, and he had to treat his low blood glucose with 15 grams of carbohydrate. He needed to add 1/2 cup of rice and 1/3 cup of beans to his lunch for more carb in the meal.

Greek. The gyro sandwich had thick pita bread as the wrap, and it was filled with lean lamb. The wrap weighed 2 ounces, so it counted as 30 grams of carbohydrate. The cucumber salad was 1 cup of cucumbers and 1/3 cup of yogurt; equal to 5 grams of carbohydrate. The lamb had no carb, so this was much below his target of 60–75 grams of carbohydrate. They checked his blood glucose log, and it showed a glucose level of 65 mg/dl after the meal. He had low blood glucose (hypoglycemia), and he had to treat it with 15 grams of carbohydrate. Examples of foods to treat low blood sugar are 1/2 cup orange juice, 1/2 cup regular carbonated beverage, or 3–4 glucose tablets. He needs to add a medium-sized piece of fruit and a glass of milk for 30 more grams of carbohydrate or a total of 62 grams of carb in the meal.

Japanese. The rice in the sushi is the source of the carbohydrate in the meal. Fortunately, he really likes sushi, so he eats enough rolls to reach his target of 60 grams of carbohydrate.

Italian. He enjoys eating the deep-dish three-cheese pizza. Each large slice of the pizza has 37 grams of carbohydrate, and he was eating 2 large slices. With a total of 90 grams of carbohydrate in this lunch, his blood glucose level 2 hours later was 160 mg/dl—higher than he wanted it. He is planning to have smaller pieces of the pizza in the future. The dietitian suggested that thin crust pizza is healthier, especially with only a regular amount of cheese and some veggies, such as mushrooms, peppers, and onions.

Keeping blood glucose records helped them see the effect of the carbohydrate on his blood glucose, so they could make adjustments in what he ate. For the days he ate Mexican or Greek, he needed to add some foods with more grams of carbohydrate. On the days he eats Chinese and Italian, he needs to adjust his servings so they are not so large, and he eats fewer grams of carbohydrate. If he didn't know what to choose from the menu, he could ask if there was nutrition information available. He could also check one of the carb counting resources in Appendix 2.

He found this exercise very useful because he could continue to eat the variety of foods that he enjoyed. But now he knew the amount of carbohydrate in each of the food items, so his blood sugar stayed within healthy ranges.

If you eat at a variety of places and you want an estimated carb count for each entrée, this type of exercise is helpful. You can do a food lab on your own or get the help of your dietitian the first time you try it, and then do it at home as your restaurant choices expand.

Fast Food

Fast food places often provide their nutrition information. If you don't see it, ask for the company's 800 number for customer service or check for their web page or information on the Internet. If you like to eat fast foods, then it is worth your time getting a copy of the nutrition information in the mail.

If information is not available, then you could use a carb reference book (Appendix 2). Here is an example of a fast food lunch. We have used our carb counting reference book and figured out that it contains the following amounts of carb:

Fast food items	Carbohydrate (g)
Bacon cheeseburger	29
Garden salad	11
Diet carbonated beverage	0
Total carbohydrate	40

This meal is not very high in carbohydrate, but the bacon cheeseburger also has 34 grams of fat and 530 calories in it. As you learned in the chapter on protein and fat, a high-fat meal could slow down the time it takes your stomach to empty. This could delay the rise in blood glucose after a meal. If you usually see a blood glucose rise within 1–2 hours after a meal, after you eat a high-fat meal, you may see a rise 3–4 hours after the meal. Use your blood glucose checks to track the effect of the food you eat.

Calculating the Carb in Your Recipes

Most people eat combination foods—such as lasagna or pizza—rather than single food items. The carb in these dishes can be trickier to count. Some examples of mixed or combination items are beef stew, hearty bean soup, or tuna noodle casserole. Your carb reference books can help with this type of food (Appendix 2). For example:

Country-style hash brown potatoes (potatoes, onions, peppers, and sausage)

Carb reference book says: 1 cup = 14 g carbohydrate
Your serving was: 2 cups = 28 g carbohydrate

Do you have a favorite recipe that does not have carbohydrate information? Start by writing down each of the ingredients. Then measure or weigh each ingredient and calculate the grams of carbohydrate in it. You can use Appendix 1 in this book or some other food reference (Appendix 2) to find the amount of carb in each ingredient. The next step is to add up all the grams of carbohydrate in the combination food. You divide the total carb by the number of servings to calculate the grams of carbohydrate in one serving. Once you've calculated the carb count of a combination food that you eat regularly, list the info in your own personal carb count book as "food/amount/carb."

Practice with a Combination Recipe

You want to find the grams of carbohydrate in your serving of this tuna noodle casserole, and you have looked up the carbohydrate grams in each ingredient.

Tuna Noodle Casserole

Ingredients	Amount	Carb (g)
Tuna	6-oz can	0
Noodles, cooked	2 cups	60
Onions, cooked	1/2 cup	5
Cream of mushroom soup	1 cup	15
Saltine crackers	6	15
Total grams of carbohydrate		95

The serving size is 1 cup, and there are 2 servings.
How much carbohydrate does 1 cup of the recipe (1 serving) contain?

Divide $\dfrac{95 \text{ g}}{2 \text{ servings}}$ = 47.5 g or round up to 48 g carbohydrate

You only need to do this calculation once and then write the carb count on the recipe card. Every time you prepare this recipe, you will know how much carbohydrate is in each serving. This takes the mystery out of what a combination or mixed-foods meal will do to your blood sugar level.

As with anything else, practice will increase your comfort level with this system. Select another one of your favorites and take it apart to calculate the grams of carbohydrate.

Your favorite combo food:

Ingredient	Amount	Carb (g)

Total grams of carbohydrate =   _____

Serving size =   _____

Number of servings in the recipe =   _____

Grams of carbohydrate in a serving =   _____

Another Meal Plan

Here is a sample meal plan based on grams of carbohydrate. Do you see how consistent it is in the amount of carbohydrate at the same meal day to day?

Carbohydrate Grams

	Mon	Tues	Wed
Breakfast	30–45	30–45	30–45
Lunch	45–60	45–60	45–60
Dinner	45–60	45–60	45–60

Read on to see how difficult it may be to get only 30–45 grams of carb at breakfast.

Take-out Breakfasts and Snack Foods

Let's look at some of the take-out foods people tend to eat and how to figure the amount of carb in them. Many of us pick up a bagel with some cream cheese on the way to work. A 1-ounce bagel is actually half of a small skinny bagel, and it has 15 g of carbohydrate. A bagel from a bakery weighs between 4–6 ounces and has between 60–75 grams of carbohydrate (or 4–5 carb choices or servings). If your carb counting target for breakfast is between 30–45 g or 2–3 servings, then the bakery bagel is too big and pushes the carb count over your target amount. You could eat half and save the other half for lunch or an afternoon snack.

Another breakfast food that people often pick up on the way to work is a baked muffin. Food references say that a 1.5-ounce muffin has 15 grams of carb. Most muffins we buy at a bakery are "mega" muffins; they weigh 6–8 ounces. They have 90–120 grams of carbohydrate or 6–8 carb choices or servings. This is way over the target of 30–45 g carb. What do you think this muffin will do to your blood sugar? We also need to look at the calories. A 1.5-ounce muffin has 100 calories, and the mega muffin has 400–500 calories. (How far will you need to walk to use up all those extra calories?)

Bagels and muffins have the same ingredients as other baked products, such as bread, biscuits, and cookies. For all these baked items, a 1-ounce serving is a 15-gram carbohydrate serving or choice. There is usually no place for you to weigh your muffin before you eat it. You could weigh a set of keys or your wallet and use them to estimate the weight of a baked product when you are on the run. If your keys or wallet weigh 4 ounces and you always have them with you, you can hold the wallet in one hand and the baked item in the other hand and make a better guess about the weight of the baked item. The weight helps you know the carbohydrate content of the item.

Compare Your Breakfast

Let's discuss another example of a work-day breakfast and compare it to a weekend restaurant breakfast.

Usual Breakfast	Weekend Breakfast
1 English muffin	4 (4-inch, 1-oz) pancakes
1/2 cup orange juice	4 Tbsp syrup
black coffee	1 cup orange juice

How many carbs are there in each breakfast? The usual breakfast has 30 g carb (2 carb choices) for the English muffin, and 15 g carb (1 carb choice) for the 1/2 cup of orange juice. This is 45 grams of carbohydrate or 3 carb choices, which is in the target range. The weekend breakfast at the restaurant has 60 g carb (4 carb choices) for the 4 pancakes, 60 g carb (4 carb choices) for the 4 tablespoons of regular syrup, and 30 g carb (2 carb choices) for the 1 cup of orange juice. The total for the weekend breakfast is 150 grams of carbohydrate or 10 carb choices or servings. See what can happen if you are not paying attention?

Lunch at a Restaurant

When you eat lunch at a restaurant, remember your target range for carbs. Soup and salad are usually considered a light lunch. But, it depends on what you put on your salad and what type of soup you have: broth based or cream based, full of beans and pasta. Let us take a look at your light lunch.

Food	Carbohydrate (g)
4 cups salad greens	8
bacon bits, egg, ham	0
1/3 cup kidney beans	15
1/3 cup of garbanzo beans	15
1 cup croutons	15
1/3 cup fat-free salad dressing	15
1 1/2 cups chicken noodle soup	<u>30</u>
Total carbohydrate	98 or
	6 1/2 carb choices

A so-called "light" lunch can easily put you out of range. How can you get this meal into your target range for carbs?

Reduce the amount of croutons to 1/2 cup and save 8 grams of carbohydrate. Reduce the salad dressing to 1 tablespoon and save 12 grams. Combine the kidney and garbanzo beans in a 1/3 cup serving and save 15 grams of carbohydrate. Only have 1 cup of the soup and save 10 grams. Your total saving is 45 grams of carbohydrate, and you're back in range. You can add 1 cup of a combination of broccoli, cauliflower, and carrots for 5 grams of carbohydrate, and you would still be within your target range without giving up too much flavor or quantity of food.

Summing Up: Tips for Restaurant Eating

All of these tips can help you become very savvy about eating out and keeping a handle on your carb count and your blood glucose levels.

- Practice at home. Once you are an expert at estimating portions at home, you will know what the servings look like on your plate anywhere, how many carbs are in the servings, and how much space on the plate the protein and fat servings take.

- Check the menu ahead of time, so you can get an idea of what you want to order. Ask your dietitian for advice. You can check a food reference book and write down grams of carbs in your favorite items. A food lab is always helpful with this, too.

- Keep a list of fast food guides handy because they provide the information on carbs for specific fast food places. You can get them from the restaurant or from their 800 customer service telephone number, or from a carb and fat reference book about fast food restaurants.

- Write down your carb target levels for each meal and snack and keep a copy with you.

10

Personal Experiences and Fine-Tuning Your Records

Now you've got some experience with carb counting under your belt, but you still have times that your blood glucose results don't seem to reflect the carbohydrate in the food you ate. Do you throw up your hands in frustration? No doubt, managing blood glucose levels can be quite frustrating. It may help to keep in mind that carb counting and managing blood glucose levels is an art—not a science. It isn't possible to keep blood glucose in perfect control all the time because blood glucose results do not reflect just the carbohydrate in foods. Blood glucose levels depend on what your blood glucose level was before you ate, the stress you're under, your physical activity (yesterday and today), your insulin resistance, how much protein and fat was part of the meal, how fast or slowly you ate, and on and on. You are a unique individual, and every time you sit down to eat, it is a new physical-chemical-emotional interaction.

The only way to get a handle on the many factors that can affect your blood glucose is to build your own "database of experiences." In other words, keep records so you can learn from a wide variety of your personal experiences. Track your individual reactions and responses to different foods and different situations. This data (or feedback) will help you shape the general guidelines to fit your diabetes and your needs.

For example, your favorite dessert is cheesecake. You have a piece at your favorite restaurant a few times a year. You are willing to check your blood glucose a couple of hours after you eat the cheesecake, and again later to check the impact of this dessert on your blood glucose level. So, what does the cheesecake do? Does it do this every time? Did you guess right about how much medication you need to cover the cheesecake (and the rest of the meal)? What will you do differently the next time?

Another example: you enjoy going for long hikes. You take a mixture of raisins and peanuts with you to eat along with a light lunch. You decrease the amount of medication you take because you know you will burn more calories and lower your blood glucose that way. So, what happens? Is this enough food or do you need a second sandwich? Did you decrease your medication too much because your blood glucose went higher than you thought it might?

Learning from your own experiences and from monitoring the reaction of your blood glucose will help you control your diabetes more than anything else. Eventually you'll be able to predict how your body will react in most of the usual daily situations. Do you think this will help give you a sense of confidence about handling your diabetes in the wide variety of experiences in your life?

Fine-Tune Your Blood Glucose Control

As you develop record-keeping skills, you can learn to see patterns in your blood glucose levels. These patterns are related to your food choices, physical activity, stress levels, and diabetes medications. Finding these patterns, identifying a reason for them, and choosing an action plan to fix them, if needed, is known as *pattern management*.

What's on the record?

You need to keep records for at least 3 days, and ideally for 7 days, to gain insight into your blood glucose patterns.

Include:

- Foods and beverages you consume
- Time of meals and snacks
- Time of blood glucose check
- Blood glucose (BG) results
- Grams of carb in meal or snack
- Type and length of physical activity
- Dose, type, and time of diabetes medications (pills or insulin)
- Workday, school day, weekend, or other type of day
- Changes such as illness, physical or emotional stress, menstruation

Finding the Patterns

In this chapter are five sample records of people with type 1 and type 2 diabetes. When you look over their records, you'll get some first-hand practice with finding the pattern and learning pattern management. The example logbooks use the same record form that is in Appendix 3.

Start with 3 days of breakfast logs to give you an idea of what is happening with your BG levels. Look for patterns of highs and lows at the same times each day. To get some practice with this process, let's meet JC, a 58-year-old male who has type 1 diabetes. The following is an example of a record of 3 days of breakfasts. JC has a target goal of 60–75 grams of carb at breakfast. His target BG level before meals is 120 mg/dl and for 2 hours after a meal, it's 160 mg/dl. We'll use a 3-step system to review JC's records on pages 118–119.

Three Steps

There is a 3-step process for fine-tuning blood glucose control. This is referred to as pattern management.

Step 1: Find the patterns. Check for blood glucose levels both above and below your target ranges. You might want to mark them with two diffferent color hi-lighters—one for high levels, one for low levels. Talk with your health care providers about your target blood glucose levels. In general, ideal blood glucose target ranges are:

Before meals:	80–120 mg/dl
After meals (1–2 hours):	160–180 mg/dl

With carb counting, checking your blood glucose 2 hours after you start to eat a meal is the only way to see what effect the diabetes medication or exercise (or both) is having on the after-meal BG level.

If your BG levels are above the target range, consider whether one or several of the following could be the cause:

- not taking the correct medication dose or the dose needs to be changed

- too much carbohydrate at the meal affects the 2 hour after-meal BG level

- more or less physical activity than planned

- physical or emotional stress

- high-protein foods

- high-fat foods

What if the BG levels are below the target range? Consider:

- delayed or missed meals or snacks

- too little carbohydrate at the meals or snacks

- diabetes medication taken incorrectly or dose needs adjustment

Step 2: Identify reasons for the highs or lows. How often are the before-meal and after-meal BG levels out of the target range? You are looking for the effect of food (mainly carbo- hyrates), diabetes medications, and physical acctivity on the BG level. Check the record for the most likely reasons that BG levels were in or out of the target range.

Step 3: Choose an action plan. Decisions about what to do are based on what you learned in step 2. Make a list of pos- sible options, such as:

- adjust the amount of carb you eat or the timing of your meal

- reduce or increase physical activity

- change diabetes medication timing or dose

Let's look at JC's record of 3 breakfasts on pages 120–121 and use the 3-step process to discuss his blood glucose patterns.

Step 1. On Monday, 2/10, the before-breakfast BG was 130 mg/dl (slightly above target). After eating 60 g carb, the 2-hour after-meal BG was 180 mg/dl. JC did no physical activity before breakfast to bring down the rise in BG, and the Monday morning stress of starting a new workweek could have raised it, too. There is no information regarding the medication dose or timing. Acarbose (Precose) should be taken right before the first bite of the meal. Also the dose starts as low as 25 mg and can worked up to 100 mg per meal, so that information needs to be added to the log.

The second day, Wednesday, 2/12, shows that even though he ate 15 grams of carb more than on Monday, the half hour of exercise and lower stress could have helped keep the after-meal BG levels lower. The weekend log shows that sleeping in, eating twice the amount of the carbo- hydrates, and getting no physical activity on Sunday, 2/16, probably contributed to the higher before- and after-meal BG levels.

Step 2. The record clearly shows the beneficial effect of exercise on JC's BG level. He even ate more carb at breakfast on the day he rode his bike.

Step 3. JC chooses to try to add a daily walk or short bike ride to his morning routine. He also decides to try a light variety of syrup instead of regular maple syrup on his pancakes to lower the number of carbs in that meal.

Meet FW   FW is newly diagnosed with type 2 diabetes and does not take diabetes medication yet. He is 45 years old. His height is 5'10" and he weights 225 pounds. His target BG levels for fasting and before meals are 80–120 and for 2 hours after meals is 160–180 mg/dl. He is not interested in a structured meal plan. He wanted to give carb counting a try, so he kept a log of 2 meals for a day to see how much carb he was eating and the effect it had on his BG levels. He did not have target carbohydrate goals because he did not know how much he was eating at meals. His record of 2 meals on one day is on page 122–123.

Step 1. His record showed that he started his day with a high BG level of 240 mg/dl. He had 124 grams of carb at breakfast and a 2-hour BG after breakfast of 308 mg/dl. His BG level before lunch was 228 mg/dl. He had 139 grams of carbohydrate at lunch and a 2-hour after-lunch BG of 318 mg/dl. This showed him that his BG levels were higher than his before- and after-meal targets.

Step 2. He was able to see a pattern in what was happening. He started his day with a high BG. His breakfast and lunch carbohydrate grams were in the 124–139 range, which was too high and that was causing the high after-meal BG levels. He did no physical activity before or after those meals to help bring the high BG levels down. This information helped him make some decisions.

Record 1. JC, male, 58 years old, ht: 5'8", wt: 208 lbs, type 2 diabetes. Target BG before meals: 120 mg/dl. 2 hrs after breakfast: 160 mg/dl.

Carbohydrate Counting and Blood Glucose Results Record

Day/Date: *Mon. 2/10, Wed. 2/12, Sun. 2/16*

Time/ meal	Diabetes medicines		Food		Carb count (choices/ grams)
	Type	Amount	Type	Amount	
8:00 a.m./ 2/10 Mon breakfast	Acarbose (Precose)	50 mg	English muffin Orange juice Margarine Coffee (black)	1 1 cup 1 tsp 1 cup	30 30 0 0 Total 60
10:00 a.m.					
8:00 a.m. Wed 2/12 breakfast	Acarbose (Precose)	50 mg	Bagel Orange juice Cream cheese Coffee black	3 oz 1 cup 1 tbsp 1 cup	45 30 0 0 Total 75
10:00 a.m.					
Sun 2/16 breakfast	Acarbose (Precose)	50 mg	Waffles, 4 inch reg. syrup Orange juice Coffee black	4 1/4 cup 1 cup 1 cup	60 60 30 0 Total 150
10:00 a.m.					
Notes about day:					

	Blood glucose results						
Fasting/before b'fast/time	After b'fast/time	Before lunch/time	After lunch/time	Before dinner/time	After dinner/time	Before bed/time	Other/time
130 (7:30 a.m.)							Stressful, start of the work week
	182						
120 (7:30 a.m.)							1/2 hr bike ride before breakfast
	158						
150 (9:30 a.m.)							Slept in late, brunch
221 noon							

Record 2. FW, male, 45 years old, ht: 5'10", wt: 225 lbs, type 2 diabetes. Target BG before meals: 80–120 mg/dl. 2 hrs after meals: 160–180 mg/dl.

Carbohydrate Counting and Blood Glucose Results Record					
Day/Date: *Monday*					
Time/ meal	Diabetes medicines		Food		Carb count (choices/ grams)
	Type	Amount	Type	Amount	
8:30 a.m./ breakfast	None		Sausage	2	0
			Biscuit, 2 oz	1	34
			Banana, med.	1	30
			Orange juice	16 oz	60
			(fast food)		Total 124
2:00 p.m. lunch	None		Cheeseburgers, Jr.	2	68
			Fries	small	33
			Chocolate chip cookies	3	38
			(fast food)		Total 139
Notes about day:					

Step 3. He decided to try to add some physical activity during the day, a 15-minute walk after lunch. (Daily exercise has the added benefit of using blood glucose even into the next day.) He discussed his carbohydrate choices with a dietitian and was willing to try a range of 80–90 carb grams per meal. Then he would keep records for 3 days (a weekend day and 2 workdays) and go through the 3-step process again to see if he needed to make further adjustments.

Blood glucose results							
Fasting/ before b'fast/ time	After b'fast/ time	Before lunch/ time	After lunch/ time	Before dinner/ time	After dinner/ time	Before bed/ time	Other/ time
240 (7:35 a.m.)	308 (10:00 a.m.)						
		228 (1:45 p.m.)	318 (3:45 p.m.)				

Meet Roberta

Roberta has learned carbohydrate counting and was keeping a record to see how she could achieve her target BG goals. She is a 60-year-old lady who lives alone and has type 2 diabetes. She has a target BG goal, fasting and before meals of 120–140 mg/dl, and a 2-hour after-meal BG target of 160–180 mg/dl. Since she lives alone, she is concerned about having hypoglycemia (low blood glucose). She was keeping this record to see how much carbohydrate she was eating, how it affected her BG level, and whether her physical activity and medication had a positive effect on her BG levels.

Record 3. Roberta, 60 years old, female, ht: 5'3", wt: 158 lbs, type 2 diabetes. Target BG fasting/pre-meal: 120–140 mg/dl. 2 hrs after meal: 160–180 mg/dl.

Carbohydrate Counting and Blood Glucose Results Record

Day/Date: *Saturday*

Time/ meal	Diabetes medicines		Food		Carb count (choices/ grams)
	Type	Amount	Type	Amount	
8:00 a.m./ breakfast	Glucovance	500 mg	Oatmeal, 1 pkg	1 cup	68
			Whole milk	1 cup	12
			Banana	1 large	25
					Total 105
12:30 p.m. lunch			Macaroni & cheese	2 cups	54
			Apple juice	1 cup	30
					Total 84
6:30 p.m. dinner	Glucovance	500 mg	Soup–chicken noodle, Campbell's	2 cups	30
			Crackers–saltine	12	12
			Canned mixed fruit cocktail, water packed	1 cup	22
					Total 68

Notes about day:

Step 1. Roberta checked for BG levels that were in or out of range. Her fasting, after breakfast, before lunch, after lunch, before dinner, and after dinner were all out of range.

Step 2. She looked for patterns. She found that she ate 105 grams of carb at breakfast and at lunch and dinner between 70–85 grams. She also noticed that a 30-minute walk before dinner helped keep the after-meal BG lower than it was after lunch with the same amount of carbo-

Blood glucose results							
Fasting/ before b'fast/ time	After b'fast/ time	Before lunch/ time	After lunch/ time	Before dinner/ time	After dinner/ time	Before bed/ time	Other/ time
174 (7:30 a.m.)	208 (10:15 a.m.)						
		196 (12:15 p.m.)	280 (1:45 p.m.)				
				180 (6:15 p.m.)	216 (7:50 p.m.)		30-minute walk before dinner

hydrate. She also noticed that her fasting BG was high—
174 mg/dl. She was on Glucovance, a combination of metformin and glyburide, but not the maximum dose for either
medication.

Step 3. She decided on a target of 80–90 carb grams per meal,
meaning a smaller breakfast and a larger dinner. This is a
middle step as these are high amounts for a small lady. She
also decided to try and walk for 30 minutes before breakfast

and before dinner. She was willing to keep logs for a few days with these changes and see what effect they had on her BG levels. She will discuss a change in medication with her health care provider, taking along these records of the changes in carbohydrate amount and physical activity.

Record 4. DT, 40-year-old female, ht: 5'5 1/2", wt: 146 lbs, type 1 diabetes. Target BG fasting/pre-meal: 80–140 mg/dl. 2 hrs after meal: 160–180 mg/dl.

Carbohydrate Counting and Blood Glucose Results Record

Day/Date: *Tuesday*

Time/ meal	Diabetes medicines		Food		Carb count (choices/ grams)
	Type	Amount	Type	Amount	
8:30 a.m./ breakfast	Lispro	5 units	Skim milk	1 cup	12
			Raisin toast	2	26
			Margarine	1	0
					Total 38
2:00 p.m. lunch	Lispro	5 units	Tuna (sandwich)	3 oz	0
			Bread	2 slices	30
			Mayonnaise	1 Tbsp	0
			Apple–large	1	30
					Total 60
5:30 p.m. dinner	Lispro	5 units	Baked potato	6 oz	30
			Chicken breast	4 oz	0
			Dinner rolls	2	30
			Banana–medium	1	30
					Total 90
9:30 p.m.	Glargine	20 units			

Notes about day:

Meet DT | DT is 40 years old, has had type 1 diabetes for 4 years, and just started on multiple daily injections of lispro before meals and glargine at bedtime. She is working with carb counting and taking the same amount of lispro with each meal.

		Blood glucose results					
Fasting/ before b'fast/ time	After b'fast/ time	Before lunch/ time	After lunch/ time	Before dinner/ time	After dinner/ time	Before bed/ time	Other/ time
Fasting 140 Pre- breakfast 8:15 a.m.	90/ 9:45 a.m.						Aerobics 1 hr after breakfast
		60/ 1:55 p.m.	120/ 4:00 p.m.				
				100/ 5:15 p.m.	180/ 7:40 p.m.		

Step 1. DT checks which BG levels are in and out of her target range, marking them with the two different colors of hi-lighter pen. Her log shows her that she has a fasting BG of 140 mg/dl. When she goes for an hour of aerobics (4–5 times a week before breakfast), her fasting BG is 70 mg/dl, showing her the direct effect of exercise on her BG level. She took 5 units of lispro before breakfast. Her carbohydrate amount at breakfast was 38 grams. She checked her BG 2 hours after breakfast, and it was 90 mg/dl.

She was going to have lunch later than usual at 2 p.m. and was concerned that she would get hypoglycemic, so she ate a chocolate candy bar with 28 grams of carbohydrate. She checked her BG before lunch, and it was 60 mg/dl. She took 5 units of lispro right before she ate 60 grams of carb. Her BG 2 hours after the meal was 120 mg/dl. Before dinner it was 100 mg/dl, and she had 90 grams of carb at dinner. Her 2-hour after-dinner BG level was 180 mg/dl. At bedtime she took her once-a-day dose of 20 units of glargine.

Step 2. Was there a pattern to her BG levels? She needs to keep records for 3 to 7 days to see a pattern. When she did, she reviewed her BG logs and saw the effect of exercise on lowering BG levels, and the effect of delayed meals on possible hypoglycemia. She noticed that lunches of 60 grams of carb worked well with 5 units of lispro. To find her insulin-to-carb ratio, she divided the 60 grams of carbohydrate by 5 units of lispro. The answer is 12, meaning that she can try taking 1 unit of lispro for every 12 grams of carbohydrate that she eats. This is called an insulin-to-carbohydrate ratio. She can try this ratio for each meal, keep BG logs before and after each meal, and collect some more data to see if it works for every meal. She may need to adjust her ratio for breakfast on the days that she does 1 hour of aerobics, because she'll probably need less insulin. Her health care provider suggests that a new ratio of 1 unit of lispro for every 15 grams of carbohydrate may work better. She did not calculate a dinner insulin:carbohydrate ratio because she was within target before and after that meal. Continuing to keep a log while she tries out the new ratio will provide information to help her make decisions about her insulin dosages.

Meet Larry

Larry is a 35-year-old construction worker with type 1 diabetes, who works Monday through Friday. He takes 2 injections of insulin a day, a combination of NPH and regular before breakfast and before dinner. He has worked with carbohydrate counting for some time. He wants to have more flexibility with his food choices, as his work and weekend time schedules are very different. He has kept a record of a typical workday. His target BG levels before meals are 110 mg/dl, and 2 hours after a meal are 140–160 mg/dl. His target carbohydrate level is 70–90 grams for each meal.

Step 1. He needs to check which BG levels are out of target range. The BG level before lunch is on the low end at 78 mg/dl; and his BG 2 hours after lunch is also lower than his target of 140–160 mg/dl. His BG before his evening meal is 150, and 200 before his bedtime snack, and 250 before bedtime, which is higher than he likes.

Step 2. He tries to find the reasons for the highs and lows. The log shows that the lunch meal was at 1:30 p.m., and breakfast was at 8 a.m., which was a long time in between. Breakfast was only 69 grams of carb, but close to the target of 70–90 grams. Also there was a lot of physical activity at work. So, there are a few variables to look at. He ate enough carbohydrate, the lunch meal was delayed, and the intensity of physical activity was high. All of these contributed to the BG of 78 mg/dl before lunch, even though he had started the day with a BG of 120 mg/dl, close to target range.

His BG 2 hours after lunch was 80 mg/dl, as he continued physical work. He had eaten his target carbohydrate at

Record 5. Larry, male, ht: 6'2", wt: 200 lbs, type 1 diabetes.
Target BG pre-meal 110 mg/dl. 2 hrs after meal 140–160 mg/dl.

Carbohydrate Counting and Blood Glucose Results Record

Day/Date: *Wednesday*

Time/ meal	Diabetes medicines		Food		Carb count (choices/ grams)
	Type	Amount	Type	Amount	
8:00 a.m.	NPH/ Regular insulin	18 N/ 5R	Egg McMuffins Orange juice	2 1 cup	54 30
					Total 84
1:30 p.m.			Cheeseburger Fries Diet soda	1 Medium 12 oz	28 43 0
					Total 71
4:00 p.m.			Chocolate chip cookie	Large	50 (from label)
6:30 p.m.	NPH/ Regular insulin	6N/5R	Steak Baked potato Corn Dinner roll	8 oz 6 oz 1 cup 2	0 30 30 30
					Total 90
9:30 p.m.			Ice cream	1 cup	30

Notes about day:

			Blood glucose results				
Fasting/ before b'fast/ time	After b'fast/ time	Before lunch/ time	After lunch/ time	Before dinner/ time	After dinner/ time	Before bed/ time	Other/ time
120 (7:50 a.m.)							Went to work Physical activity
		78 (1:25 p.m.)					
			80 (3:30 p.m.)				
							Worked construction
				150 (6:20 p.m.)			Watched TV
					200 (8:30 p.m.)	250 (11:00 p.m.)	Watched TV

his lunch meal, but his 2-hour BG of 80 after the lunch meal was much lower than his target BG of 140–150 mg/dl after a meal. This could have been due to the intensity of the physical activity at work. He probably needs to eat more carb at breakfast and lunch. The pattern during the day was BG levels on the low side compared to his targets for the day. However, his evening BG levels were higher than his target, perhaps from the carbohydrate in the cookie he ate mid-afternoon and from dinner and the ice cream before bedtime.

Step 3. He was interested in considering some changes based on what he had learned in steps 1 and 2. He discussed with his health care provider the possibility of taking more injections matched to his meals to increase his flexibility, so he could eat on an irregular schedule, have more physical activity, and still meet his target BG goals. He was interested in moving on to using insulin-to-carbohydrate ratios. One option for the high evening BG levels and fasting morning BG would be to split his evening NPH and regular dose into 2 shots, take the regular with his evening meal and the NPH at bedtime. He could try his usual dose of 5 units of regular before the evening meal, and keep the carbohydrate within his target of 70–90 grams. To figure his insulin:carb ratio, he divides 80 grams of carbohydrate by the 5 units of regular. This gives an answer of 16, meaning he will use 1 unit of regular for every 16 grams of carbohydrate that he eats. This is a place for him to start. He will see if it is working by recording before-meal and 2 hour after-meal BG levels for 3 to 7 days to see if they are in target range. If it works for dinner, he can try it for all his meals and snacks.

Don't go too low

As you looked at the records, you probably noticed some low BG levels. Hypoglycemia, or BG levels that are 70 mg/dl or lower, is a condition that you want to avoid.

But the more you bring your blood glucose levels closer to normal, the more chances you might slip too low. When your blood glucose is too low your thinking and coordination are impaired. In Larry's case, this could cause an accident on the job. If your blood glucose goes too low, you could lose consciousness. To avoid hypoglycemia, take care to eat your target amount of carb at regular meals and snacks and get moderate amounts of exercise. If you take diabetes medications, be sure you are taking the correct dose at the proper time. If you exercise more than usual, eat more carb or adjust your medication dose. Even then, hypoglycemia can surprise you. Try to plan so you can avoid it, and be ready to deal with it, if it happens.

What can cause hypoglycemia?

1. Too much insulin, or sulfonylureas, Prandin, Glucovance, or Starlix.
2. A meal or snack not eaten on time, or not enough carb at a meal or snack.
3. Increased physical activity or exercise but no reduction in the amount of insulin or medication or not eating a snack when you need one.

What are the symptoms of hypoglycemia?

Common symptoms of low blood glucose are:

- shakiness

- sweating

- feeling disoriented or dizzy

- headache

Many people have their own individual symptoms. You need to be familiar with your own symptoms of low blood glucose and tell them to your family, friends, and co-workers, so they can recognize it, too. Also tell them what to do to help you. When you are experiencing low blood glucose levels, you need help, and you may not be able to explain it then.

What do you do for low blood glucose?

An easy way to remember what to do is the rule of 15/15. Treat hypoglycemia with 15 grams of carbohydrate, and wait 15 minutes. Check your BG level and make sure it has come up. If it is still less than 70 mg/dl, then repeat the 15/15. Examples of 15 grams of carbohydrate are 4–6 ounces of fruit juice, 4–6 ounces of regular soda (not diet), 6 small hard candies, glucose tablets (see the label for the dose), and glucose gel (see the label for the dose).

Always carry some source of glucose with you. You can carry glucose tablets in your purse, pocket, briefcase, backpack, console of your car, and keep them in the bedside table. If you feel that your blood glucose level is already slipping too low, treat first and then check your BG level.

Some people who have had type 1 diabetes for years or who have had many episodes of low blood glucose may develop "hypoglycemia unawareness." This means that they get low blood sugar, but they don't get any symptoms. If this happens to you, protect yourself by doing frequent BG checks and ask your diabetes care provider for training in BG awareness. You don't want to go so low that you pass out. Your family, friends, and co-workers should also be aware of this and know how to use glucagon to bring your blood glucose level back up if you are unconscious. Glucagon is a prescription item and can be obtained with a prescription from your health care provider.

Do not drive until you have checked your BG to make sure it is in a safe range. Always carry a soda, candy, or glucose tablets where you can reach them in your car.

Checks and Records

Checking your blood glucose levels frequently can help you limit low blood sugars. Keeping a record so that you can see whether there is a pattern to the "lows" can help you head off hypoglycemia. In this and in many ways, your records can provide you with information that can keep you on an even keel with diabetes, thereby improving your health and your quality of life. Record keeping is an investment of time that can pay big dividends.

Ready, Willing, and Able to Progress?

If you have mastered basic carb counting, and you answer YES to most of the questions below, you are probably ready for advanced carb counting.

1. You cannot achieve your target blood glucose levels with basic carb counting.

☐ yes   ☐ no

You need more detailed food and blood glucose records to decide how much rapid- or short-acting insulin to take before meals. This can help you achieve your target blood glucose and HbA$_{1c}$ levels.

2. It is too difficult for you to eat similar amounts of carbohydrate at your meals and snacks each day. Because of your lifestyle and eating habits, you want more flexibility in the amount of carbohydrate you eat at meals and snacks.

☐ yes   ☐ no

3. You can (and are willing to) do the math to make adjustments in the amount of medication (insulin) to take based on your insulin-to-carbohydrate ratio and the amount of carbohydrate you eat.

☐ yes   ☐ no

4. You are willing and able to check your blood glucose levels at least 4 times each day in order to figure the amount of medication (insulin) to take based on the amount of carbohydrate you will eat.

☐ yes ☐ no

5. You are willing to take the time to analyze your blood glucose results and review patterns and other factors to continue to fine-tune your diabetes plan.

☐ yes ☐ no

6. You have a diabetes care provider who is willing and able to help you practice advanced carb counting.

☐ yes ☐ no

Meet Bob

Bob has had diabetes for about 17 years. He is 67 now and has been retired for two years from his career as an engineer. For the first 10 or so years he had diabetes, he really didn't pay much attention to it other than taking his diabetes pills. He monitored his blood glucose just when he thought it might be too high, but not regularly. He didn't pay too much attention to what he was eating and when. Unfortunately, Bob recently began seeing spots in one of his eyes. It was diagnosed as diabetic retinopathy, and he had some laser surgery to delay its further progression. This made Bob realize that he had better start paying more attention to his diabetes if he wants to keep seeing and keep other parts of his body healthy. He has been monitoring his blood glucose levels more often and realizes that they are often over 200 mg/dl. His doctor recently suggested that, along with the diabetes pills, he should take quick-acting insulin just before he eats his meals. His doctor also suggested that he have a few sessions with a dietitian to learn how to decide how much insulin he needs to take based on what he chooses to eat.

At his first visit, he and the dietitian talked about what Bob was willing to do to take care of his diabetes. The dietitian let Bob know that making decisions about how much insulin to take before meals takes effort and some mathematics. Since Bob now has a bit of time on his hands, he decided he wants to try this method. The dietitian told Bob that they would start with the basics about carbohydrates and determine how much carbohydrate he wants and needs at each of his meals. She explained how the amount of rapid-acting insulin he takes will be determined by two things—what Bob's blood glucose is before his meal and what he plans to eat. The dietitian told Bob that he should return for several visits to make sure he understands how to do this and to fine-tune his insulin-to-carbohydrate ratio (the amount of carbohydrate that can be covered by 1 unit of rapid-acting insulin) (Read more about fine-tuning your diabetes control and these ratios in chapter 12.)

Bob left the dietitian's office with a better understanding of what foods contain carbohydrate. He also has a basic plan for how many carb choices or grams of carbohydrate he needs at breakfast, lunch, and dinner. In addition, Bob knows that he will start using an insulin-to-carbohydrate ratio of 1:15 or 1 unit of rapid-acting insulin to cover each 15 grams of carbohydrate. The key now is to follow this meal plan carefully, which includes weighing and measuring his foods for awhile and monitoring his blood glucose both before and after his meals. Checking his blood glucose is the only way to fine-tune his insulin-to-carbohydrate ratio so it works for him. Before leaving, Bob makes the next appointment with the dietitian in 2 weeks. She asks him to remember to bring in his food and blood glucose records for the visit. She also encourages him to bring in food labels from foods he usually eats and a list of the foods he typically eats when he dines out. They will figure out how he can fit these foods into his carbohydrate counting plan, too.

12

Advanced Carb Counting
Using Insulin-to-Carbohydrate Ratios

Advanced carb counting is most appropriate for people who have decided that they are willing to do what it takes to achieve a tighter level of blood glucose control—counting carbs, checking blood glucose often, exercising, keeping good records, and making daily decisions about their diabetes care from the information in their records. At the advanced level, you and your provider use these records to create your personal formula for figuring how much insulin to take to "cover" the carbohydrate in your meal—your insulin:carbohydrate ratio. Most people who do advanced carb counting are taking insulin. They are either taking multiple daily injections (three or more shots a day) or using an insulin pump. This isn't exclusive to people with type 1 diabetes. Many people who have had type 2 for years take insulin or a combination of oral medications and insulin in order to achieve tight control. While the dosages of several rapid-acting pills can be adjusted, most pills cannot be adjusted to cover changes in the amount of carbohydrate in an individual meal.

As you move forward, please recognize that advanced carb counting and the adjustment of diabetes medications is not a do-it-yourself activity. The body is very complex, and each person with diabetes is unique. If you believe that advanced carb counting and the related adjusting of your medications is for you, we encourage you to find and work closely with diabetes care providers who are knowledgeable about this type of diabetes management. Find providers who are willing to give you the time you need as you develop and apply the ratios as well as work with you to fine-tune your control and make adjustments as your diabetes and your lifestyle change.

A New Vocabulary

You'll hear certain words and phrases often when you enter the world of advanced carb counting. Let's define these first.

Basal insulin. The pancreas of a person who does not have diabetes puts out about 1 unit of insulin per hour, whether or not any food is eaten. This is simply the amount of insulin the body needs hour to hour to keep functioning properly and to supply glucose to the cells. If you take insulin, *basal insulin* is what you need to keep your blood sugar level in control regardless of whether you eat any food. Another term used for basal insulin is *background insulin.*

Basal insulin is either intermediate-acting insulin (NPH or Lente) or long-acting insulin (Ultralente or glargine [Lantus]). Look at Figures 12-1 and 12-2 to see the action curves of the different types of insulin. People on an insulin pump set a basal rate of rapid- or short-acting insulin to be infused over 24 hours.

Establishing the amount of basal insulin that you need is not simple. For example, we know that for many people, blood sugar goes up before they wake due to a rise in hormones at that time of day. This is called the *dawn phenomenon* and often requires more insulin. We know that some people have a tendency to get low blood sugars during the night, but not every night. All this is to say that there are many variables to consider as you fine-tune your background insulin. Generally, about 50% of your total insulin intake in 24 hours will be your basal insulin, but you might

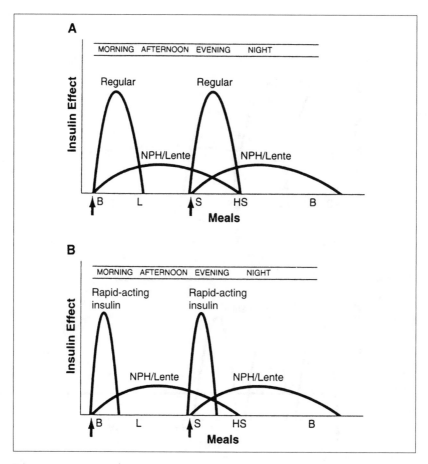

Figure 1 (**A**) Short-acting and intermediate-acting insulin. (**B**) Rapid-acting and intermediate-acting insulin. (B = breakfast, L = lunch, S = supper, HS = evening snack, B = bedtime)

find you need as little as 45% or as much as 60%. You do not use insulin:carb ratios to determine basal insulin doses.

Bolus insulin. When people who don't have diabetes eat food, their bodies automatically put the amount of insulin they need into the bloodstream to keep blood sugar under about 140 mg/dl. This amount of insulin lowers blood sugar rapidly. *Bolus insulin* is the amount of rapid- or short-acting

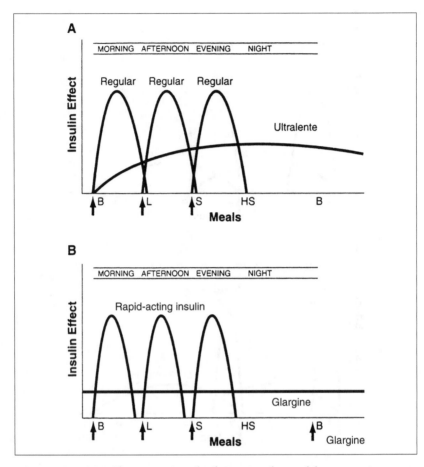

Figure 2 (**A**) Short-acting before meals and long-acting insulin in the morning. (**B**) Rapid-acting with meals and glargine at bedtime.
(B = breakfast, L = lunch, S = supper, HS = evening snack, B = bedtime)

insulin that you need to "cover" the amount of food—especially carbohydrate—that you eat. Bolus insulin is the insulin you need to bring your blood sugar back to target pre-meal levels within about 3 hours after beginning a meal. Bolus insulin can account for as little as 40% of the total daily insulin dose or as much as 55%. You do use your insulin:carb ratio to calculate your bolus insulin doses.

Insulin:carb ratio. An insulin-to-carbohydrate ratio tells you the amount of rapid-acting insulin you need to "cover" the amount of carbohydrate you eat to bring your after-meal blood sugar back to target levels. Advanced carb counting helps you develop an insulin:carb ratio that works best for you. Many people begin with an insulin:carb ratio of 1:15. This means that you need 1 unit of rapid- or short-acting insulin for every 15 grams of carbohydrate you eat.

For example: your meal has 72 g of carb in it. To find out how much insulin you need to take to cover it, you divide the grams of carb in the meal by the number of carbs covered by 1 unit of insulin.

$$\frac{72\ g}{15\ g} = 4.8 \text{ or round up to } 5$$

You need to take 5 units of rapid- or short-acting insulin to cover the carbohydrate in this meal. When you use insulin:carb ratios to figure your bolus insulin doses, you can be much more flexible about what and how much you eat—and when you eat, too.

People who are sensitive to insulin—meaning that small amounts of insulin lower their blood sugar rapidly—might need a higher insulin:carb ratio, such as 1:20. And on the other hand, people who are insensitive to insulin—meaning it takes a lot of insulin to lower their blood sugar—might need a lower insulin:carb ratio, such as 1:10. To make things even more interesting, you might find that you need to use different insulin:carb ratios at different times of day. For example, some people who eat the same amount of carb at breakfast, lunch, and dinner need more insulin in the morning than they do at lunch or dinner.

Postprandial blood glucose (PPG). Postprandial blood glucose is the blood glucose level after you eat. In advanced carb counting, checking your PPG is the only way to see how well your bolus doses and your insulin:carb ratio are working. Most clinicians agree that PPG is defined as the blood sugar level 2 hours after the start of a meal. Until further research helps us set guidelines for PPG, diabetes care providers generally agree that the target for PPG is ≤160 mg/dl.

Multiple daily injections (MDI). People who want to control their blood glucose levels closely take multiple daily insulin injections—three or more shots per day. Generally, people on MDI take basal insulin in two shots a day of intermediate-acting insulin—one before breakfast and one before bed. But some people take their basal insulin as one injection of long-acting insulin before bed if they use insulin glargine. Everyone on MDI takes bolus injections of rapid- or short-acting insulin before each meal and possibly before large snacks to control blood sugar. You use your insulin:carb ratio to determine the dose of rapid- or short-acting insulin that you need to cover meals.

Insulin pump. The type of insulin pump available today is called an "open-loop pump." A "closed-loop pump" would automatically check your blood sugar and automatically give you the amount of insulin you need, but they haven't been perfected yet. With the open-loop pump, you check your blood sugar and decide how much insulin you need—both basal and bolus. You only use rapid- or short-acting insulin in the pump.

An insulin pump is a small device about the size of a pager. Very thin plastic tubing runs from the syringe in the pump to a very fine needle or plastic tube that is inserted under the skin in the abdomen or another place that is comfortable for you. Pumps can hold up to 300 units of insulin. With assistance from your pump trainer and diabetes care providers, you "program" the pump to provide both basal and bolus insulin. Basal insulin is provided in continuous tiny amounts over 24 hours. You can adjust the basal amount in various ways with most pumps to get more or less basal insulin during a 24-hour period. You decide how much bolus insulin to take by checking your pre-meal blood sugar and the amount of carb you decide to eat. All in all, the insulin pump delivers insulin in a way that more closely mimics the way a normal pancreas does. This is one reason most people who start using a pump are able to decrease the amount of insulin they take by about 20%.

How to Find Your Insulin:Carb Ratio

Now that you've got some advanced carb counting terms under your belt, let's move on to ways to determine your own insulin:carb ratios. As a word of caution, always be conservative. You don't want to take too much insulin because you don't want your blood sugar to go too low. Work out your insulin:carb ratios with the advice of your diabetes care provider.

Method #1: Using your food diary and blood glucose records

You can use the food and blood glucose record you find in Appendix 3 or a form that you have developed. You need a record of several days but best is a whole week to determine your insulin:carb ratio. Be sure to track the grams of carb you eat, the amount of rapid- or short-acting insulin you take before the meal, and your blood glucose results. Note whenever your blood glucose is too high or too low. It is helpful to do more blood glucose checks during this phase— both before you eat and 2 hours after you start eating (PPG). All this information will help you establish a more precise insulin:carb ratio. While you're compiling your daily records, it is a good idea to try and keep your carb grams and the amount of activity you do as consistent as possible.

Look at your records. For each meal or snack you ate, divide the total grams of carb by the number of units of rapid- or short-acting that insulin you took to achieve your target blood glucose level. You might well find that you need different insulin:carb ratios for different times of the day. You might also find that you need different amounts of insulin for certain foods or meals, such as pizza, a high-protein and high-fat meal, or for prolonged meals, such as a buffet dinner party.

Example: Look first at breakfasts. You see that generally you eat about 60 grams of carb, and you take about 4 units of rapid-acting insulin. This amount of insulin seems to get you back to your pre-meal target blood sugar within three hours. That's good. To find a breakfast insulin:carb ratio, you divide 60 g carb by 4 units insulin. The answer is 15 or 1 unit of insulin for every 15 grams of carbohydrate—an insulin:carb ratio of 1:15.

Method #1 will work for you if your blood sugar level is generally within your targets both before and after eating. If you are not near your targets, this method will not be as helpful because the amount of insulin you are taking is not achieving good blood sugar control. Method #2 might work better as a starting point.

Method #2: The rule of 500

We'll introduce you to two "rules" in this chapter that have no formal research to support them. They are, however, used by many diabetes care providers and their patients. The first—the rule of 500—can be used to calculate your starting insulin:carb ratios. The second—the rule of 1500—helps you figure out how much additional insulin to take when your blood glucose level is higher than your target level before the meal.

The 500 rule is useful in determining your initial insulin:carb ratio if you take rapid-acting insulin. Some clinicians use 450 to calculate the insulin:carb ratio if you take short-acting insulin.

Here's how to use it. Divide the number 500 by your total daily dose of insulin. You find your total daily dose by adding all the insulin you take in 24 hours—both short and long acting. If your total daily insulin dose is 42 units, divide 500 by 42. The answer is the number of grams of carb covered by 1 unit of rapid-acting insulin.

Example:

Your total daily insulin dose is 42 units.
500 divided by 42 = 12

Your insulin:carb ratio is 1:12.
You take 1 unit of insulin for every 12 g carbohydrate in the meal or snack.

Check it out. Did you get the same insulin:carb ratio using method #1 that you got with this method? Are they close or far apart? The only way to check whether the insulin:carb ratio works for you is to use it and check you blood glucose levels frequently. You will soon learn whether it works for you or you will have the information to figure a new insulin:carb ratio that should be more effective for you.

The insulin pump companies also provide guidelines for how to choose the beginning insulin:carb ratios based on a person's weight. Again, this is a way to get you started. Your records will help you zero in on the ratios that work best for you.

Now, you have an insulin:carb ratio or 1:12. Your breakfast has 60 g carb in it. How much insulin are you going to take to cover the carb in the meal? Divide the total carb in the meal by the number of carb grams one unit of insulin will cover.

$$\frac{60}{12} = 5 \text{ units of insulin}$$

You will take 5 units of insulin to cover your 60 g carb meal.

Correcting High Blood Glucose Before a Meal: The Rule of 1500

Now, you have used your insulin:carb ratio to figure how much insulin to take to cover the carb in the meal, but you check your blood sugar before you eat, and it's higher than your pre-meal target. What do you do? You have a second calculation to make to find out how much additional insulin you need to get your blood sugar back to your target level. This is a different ratio that tells you how much 1 unit of insulin lowers your blood glucose level. It is called a *correction factor* or *insulin sensitivity factor*. The amount of insulin you need to take depends on how sensitive you are to the insulin. As long as you know how to calculate yours and how to use it correctly, it doesn't matter what you call it.

The rule of 1500 is a method to calculate how much 1 unit of rapid- or short-acting insulin lowers your blood sugar. This rule was developed by Dr. Paul Davidson, in Atlanta, Georgia.

Here's how it works. As with the rule of 500, you need to figure your total daily dose of insulin. That's all the insulin you take during the course of an average day. Then divide 1500 by your total daily dose of insulin to find your correction factor. If your total daily dose is 35, you divide 1500 by 35 to find your correction factor is 43. This means that 1 unit of insulin lowers your blood glucose by 43 mg/dl.

Example:

$$\frac{1500}{35 \text{ (total daily dose)}} = 43 \text{ (correction factor)}$$

1 unit of insulin will lower your blood sugar by 43 mg/dl.
Your ratio is 1:43.

Some clinicians find that using the number 1800 is more accurate for people who take rapid-acting insulin or have insulin sensitivity.

Now you have a correction factor, what do you do with it? Let's try an example.

You check your blood glucose before dinner, and it is 225 mg/dl. Your target before-meal blood sugar level is 100 mg/dl.

To find out how much you need to lower your blood sugar to get to the target, you subtract the target level from the actual blood sugar.

$$
\begin{array}{r}
225 \text{ (actual blood sugar)} \\
-100 \text{ (target pre-meal blood sugar)} \\
\hline
125 \text{ mg/dl}
\end{array}
$$

You need to lower your blood sugar by 125. If you take 1 unit of insulin to lower your blood sugar by 43 mg/dl, how many units of insulin do you need to lower it by 125 mg/dl?

Divide 125 by 43.

$$\frac{125}{43 \text{ (correction factor)}} = 2.9 \text{ or round up to 3 units of insulin}$$

If your before-meal target is a range of 80–120 mg/dl, then you can select a number within that range to use in your calculations. You may want to use the midpoint of 100 or the high end of 120. The important thing to remember while you are finding out what correction factor works best for you is not to overcorrect so that you go too low.

Figuring Your Insulin Dose

Using the two "rules" in the previous examples, we have found that you need 5 units of insulin to cover the 60 g of carbohydrate in your breakfast. You also need 3 units of insulin to bring your blood sugar back to your pre-meal target. So, to figure how much rapid- or short-acting insulin to take, you add the two results.

5 units for the meal
3 units to correct
8 units of insulin

Here's another opportunity for you to practice.

Example:

Pre-meal blood sugar is 175
Target pre-meal blood sugar is 120
Correction factor is 1 unit to lower blood sugar
50 points
Amount of carb in meal is 69 grams
Insulin:carb ratio is 1:15

175 (actual blood sugar)
−120 (target pre-meal blood sugar)
55

You need to lower your blood sugar by 55 mg/dl

$$\frac{55}{50 \text{ (correction factor)}} = 1 \text{ unit of insulin}$$

You need to take 1 additional unit of insulin to correct the too-high blood sugar.

Insulin:carb ratio is 1:15 for this meal.

$$\frac{69 \text{ g carb}}{15} = 4.6 \text{ or round up to 5 units of insulin}$$

You add the correction insulin to the meal insulin.

1 unit
+ 5 units
6 units

You take 6 units of pre-meal bolus insulin.

It's important to look at the patterns of your blood sugar. If day after day you have to use one or several units of insulin to correct your blood glucose level before a meal, then you either need more basal insulin in the time leading up to that meal or you need to increase the bolus insulin for the previous meal. Use the information you gain from having to use correction factors to make finer adjustments to your insulin doses and be within your target ranges all day long.

What about Pre-Meal Lows?

If your blood sugar before the meal is lower than your target level, then you don't want it to go any lower. You have three options:

1. **Eat more carbohydrate at the meal.** In the example on page 150, you could add another 15 grams of carb to the 69 grams in the meal but not take any more insulin.
2. **Take less insulin.** Using the same example, you would subtract 1 unit of insulin from the mealtime dose and only take 4 units of insulin for the 69 grams of carb.
3. **Give the carb a "running start."** Take the 5 units of insulin to cover the carb but give the carb a "running start" by delaying the pre-meal bolus a few minutes until your blood sugar level is rising from the food you're eating.

With experimentation you will learn whether one way works better than another for you. In these situations, you must be alert for signs of hypoglycemia and treat it as soon as it is coming on.

If you have frequent high or low pre-meal blood sugar levels, then you need to check your basal dose, too. Work with your diabetes care providers to help you make the needed adjustments to get your numbers closer to targets.

Common Questions about Advanced Carb Counting

How do you know how much insulin you need?
There is no simple answer to this question. One way to get an estimate of your insulin needs is to allow 0.14 to 0.23 units of insulin per pound of body weight. It is best to be conservative and only increase the insulin dosage as your blood sugar records indicate you need to. This helps you avoid having low blood sugar. However, this estimate will not work for everyone. People with type 1 diabetes can be insulin sensitive, so they might need less insulin. People with type 2 often have some insulin resistance, and they need more insulin to control blood sugar levels. Insulin needs can change as you move through different phases of your life or change your lifestyle. For example, adolescents have surging hormones, which can cause higher than usual insulin needs, and women have different insulin needs in different phases of their menstrual cycle or in different trimesters of pregnancy. A man in retirement who takes up a sport such as bicycling and gets into long-distance rides will have different insulin needs than he did before.

How often do you have to change the correction factor or figure a new insulin:carb ratio?
Any time your total daily dose changes beyond just a couple of units up or down, review your ratios and correction factors and make sure they are still working well for you. Are you running into unexpected lows? You only need to change your correction factor or insulin:carb ratio when you have a significant change in your total daily insulin dose or in your lifestyle. For example, you have not been physically active, but you have decided to begin a walking program 3 days a week. You may have to lower your insulin dose several times over the following weeks as your body adjusts to the effect of the exercise on your blood glucose levels. This is the time to consider a change in your correction factor or insulin:carb ratio. Examine your blood sugar

records to see what is happening. You may find that you need to use different factors on activity and non-activity days. As you lose weight over the next year from regular exercise, you may well have to adjust your correction factor and ratios again.

How do you keep all these factors and guidelines straight?
The first thing to do is write down your correction factor and your insulin:carb ratio(s). Keep them with your insulin kit, in your calendar or wallet, or post them on the refrigerator. Make sure they are where you need them when you need them. Certainly it won't take long to commit them to memory, but then they might change. Don't leave yourself guessing.

How do you do all the math?
It is important to have a calculator with you or available to you. A calculator helps with the math as you practice using advanced carb counting. Discuss how to use your insulin:carb ratios and your correction factor with your health care provider until you feel comfortable using them on your own.

What is the difference between using rapid-acting insulin and short-acting insulin?
Rapid-acting insulin works more quickly than short-acting regular insulin, so its action is more likely to coincide with the rise in blood sugar from the food you've eaten. As the carb is raising blood sugar, the rapid-acting insulin is beginning to lower blood sugar. Regular insulin doesn't peak until 3–4 hours after the meal and can miss the mark, so to speak. If you think rapid-acting insulin would work better for you, talk to your diabetes care provider. Never make this switch on your own. Here are a few factors for you and your provider to consider:

- If you are on MDI taking regular with meals but plan to switch to rapid-acting insulin before meals, then your intermediate- or long-acting insulin may need to be increased slightly to continue to control your blood sugar between meals. Because regular insulin lasts longer, it also has some basal action, but rapid-acting insulin does not.

- If your blood sugar is in your target range before you switch from regular to rapid-acting insulin, decrease your rapid-acting insulin dose by 20% as compared to the dose of regular. This is because rapid-acting insulin works more efficiently than regular insulin.

- When you have made this switch, check your blood sugar 2 hours after starting meals for several days. This will help you see how the rapid-acting insulin dose is working.

- If your blood glucose level is higher than your target level before meals (or in-between meals), then you could try a unit for unit switch from regular to rapid-acting insulin. But, if your morning fasting blood glucose is above your target range, you need to bring it within target range for at least 3 days before you make a switch from regular to rapid-acting insulin.

- If your target ranges are eluding you, check before- and after-meal blood glucose levels often to get a picture of what is happening.

Do you need to eat snacks on a MDI or insulin pump?
You can snack less often using MDI or an insulin pump, or you may be able to omit snacks, particularly if you use rapid-acting insulin. Remember that rapid-acting insulin works with the rise of blood sugar from the meal and is gone from the body within several hours. So, if you don't want to eat snacks, this may work for you. If you want to eat snacks because you enjoy them or find that they help you control your blood sugar better, then you need to determine—with blood sugar checks—whether you need more insulin. See chapter 4.

For snacks in-between meals or a bedtime snack do you need to take more insulin?
If you take rapid-acting insulin, you may need to take some to cover an in-between meal snack or a bedtime snack, particularly if those snacks are large. If you have different insulin:carb ratios for different meals, try using the ratio for the meal closest to the snack. If you take regular insulin, it usually is working hardest within 2–3 hours of being injected. So you may not need extra insulin because it will still be working when you've eaten your snack. Again checking blood glucose levels is the way to decide what works for you and what doesn't.

How does a high-fat or high-protein meal affect the rise in blood sugar? How does pizza impact blood sugar? How does grazing at a cocktail party for several hours impact blood sugar?
As we discussed in chapter 6, the impact of high-fat, high-protein meals may be different for people with type 1 diabetes than for people with insulin resistant type 2 diabetes. Here's a starting point. If you take rapid- or short-acting insulin, take the insulin based on your blood sugar level and insulin:carb ratio. Then check your blood glucose 2 to 3 hours after the meal to see if it is in your target range. A high-fat or high-fat, high-protein meal, such as prime rib, may delay stomach emptying and the rise in blood sugar from 2 hours after the start of the meal to 3 to 5 hours after the start of the meal. If you take rapid-acting insulin, it may peak before your blood sugar peaks, and you end up with hypoglycemia. To prevent this, some people take rapid-acting insulin after a high-fat meal, rather than before, or split the dose and take half before and half after the meal. Clearly, checking your blood sugar level is the only way you will know the effect of these foods on you.

Pizza is a food that causes blood sugar to rise high in some people. Count the carbs in the serving you eat, use your insulin:carb ratio, and check 2 hours later to see what it does to your blood sugar levels. If there is a lot of meat and cheese on the pizza, check your blood sugar again 3 to 5 hours after starting the meal. Keep close records the next time you eat pizza, too. This is important information for you—and you'll use it every time you want to eat pizza.

Using an insulin pump allows you various ways of managing these situations. You can calculate the bolus insulin dose for the entire meal, and take 2/3 the dose at the start of the meal. Then, 2–3 hours later check your blood glucose and, depending on the level, take the rest of the bolus dose. Most pumps have an option that lets you extend the bolus dose of insulin over several hours. This works well with meals that raise blood sugar more slowly and meals that extend over a longer than usual period of time, such as thanksgiving or large dinner parties.

Should you adjust the amount of rapid- or short-acting insulin you take for a high-fiber meal?
Yes, if a food or meal has 5 grams or more of fiber, subtract the grams of fiber from the total grams of carbohydrate in the meal. This is because the fiber part of the total carbohydrate is, for the most part, not digested and not absorbed as glucose. Calculate how much rapid- or short-acting insulin to take based on the amount of carb in the meal, minus the grams of dietary fiber.

Here is an example of a high fiber breakfast:

Food	Fiber	Carb
1 cup high fiber cereal	6 g	32 g
1 slice whole-grain bread	3 g	12 g
1 cup low-fat milk	0 g	12 g
1 1/4 cup strawberries	2 g	15 g
Total	11 g	71 g

Subtract the 11 grams of fiber from the 71 grams of carbohydrate, and figure your insulin dose on 60 g carb. Based on an insulin:carb ratio of 1:15, the insulin dose would be:

$$\frac{60}{15} = 4 \text{ units of insulin}$$

Should you adjust the amount of rapid- or short-acting insulin for alcohol?
Alcohol tends to lower blood sugar levels, so you do not need additional insulin to cover it. In fact, alcohol can lower blood sugar several hours after you drink it, so you may want to check your blood sugar then, too. As most people drink alcohol in the evening, you may need to eat a bedtime snack or have a bigger snack than you usually do. Always eat food when you have alcohol. If you have a mixed drink with fruit juice or a carbohydrate-containing beverage, check the amount of carbohydrate in the drink and add it to the total carb in the meal, and then calculate your insulin based on your insulin:carb ratio. If you check your blood sugar before and after you drink the alcoholic beverage (and eat the meal), you can get a better idea of its effect on your blood sugar level.

Less frequently, alcohol can cause a rise in blood sugar. This is due to the carbohydrate in some alcoholic beverages, such as beer and sweet wine, or the carbohydrate from a mixer, such as orange juice or regular cola. So, if you drink these kinds of alcoholic beverages with a meal when your diabetes medications are not working to lower blood sugar, your blood sugar may rise.

What do you do when there is a variation in blood glucose levels but no specific pattern?
Look for changes in your daily schedule, such as missed meals or variable amounts of exercise. These will throw your blood glucose levels off and make you think that your insulin:carb ratio isn't working. Check your log, do you find:

- missed meals or snacks   yes   no

- variable exercise   yes   no

- stress   yes   no

▪ varied eating schedule*	yes	no
▪ different amount of carbs	yes	no

If you answer yes to several or all of these, then do you also find in your log:

▪ insulin doses that change often	yes	no
▪ frequent hypoglycemia	yes	no
▪ frequent hyperglycemia	yes	no

*Does not matter if you are on a pump and the basal rate is adjusted appropriately.

There is a connection between the changes in the first list and the results in the second list. Let's practice sleuthing. Your fasting blood glucose is in your target range, and you are having a pattern of high blood glucose levels related to a specific meal. The meal is usually one you eat at a restaurant or a friend's home or consists of foods that you have not eaten in the past.

Your insulin:carb ratio is 1 unit of rapid-acting insulin for every 15 grams of carb, and you have a target range of 75 grams of carb. You take 5 units to cover the meal based on your insulin:carb ratio, but your blood glucose is high after that meal. You could have miscalculated the carbs in the meal. If your estimate of the carbs is off, do a review of weighing and measuring your servings or the contents of the meal to get back on track.

You eat out at a favorite restaurant and order a specific item you enjoy and your after-meal blood glucose levels are higher than your target. Record the grams of carb that you estimate in the meal and how many units you took to cover it. After you've had the meal several different times, check your log for how many units of insulin you took to cover the meal and what your blood glucose was after the meal, and you will have a good idea of how much insulin you need to take the next time. Another option is to purchase the meal, take it home, and weigh and measure the contents. Look up the carb content of the ingredients and then total the carb grams. This gives you a number to work with next time you have this meal.

There is no substitute for blood glucose checks and keeping detailed records to sort out the changes in patterns. Discuss the changes and possible causes and solutions with your health care provider.

How does physical activity affect your blood glucose levels?
Exercise lowers blood glucose, so you have to reduce your insulin dose or eat more carbohydrate to compensate. This is to prevent hypoglycemia. For safety, always try to have your blood glucose levels between 90–150 mg/dl while exercising. After exercise, your blood sugar should not drop below 70 mg/dl. You may need to do blood glucose checks before and after exercise whenever the exercise lasts 45 minutes or more. If the exercise is long and intense, check your blood glucose over the next 24–36 hours, because it can continue to fall for that length of time. Check with your diabetes care provider about adjusting basal insulin doses that apply during and after periods of physical activity.

What about stress?
Stress is a normal part of life, but it can interfere with blood glucose control. Your appetite, how well you rest, and how much physical activity you get may all change when you are under stress. Sleep may be inadequate during times of stress. Even though it would be the best thing for you, you may not get enough physical activity to promote relaxation during stressful times. This may be a time that blood glucose levels go up and down unpredictably, and this can be related to not having your regular routine. Stress also interferes with blood glucose control by the release of certain hormones. These hormones can cause your body to release additional glucose into your bloodstream and can also interfere with the action of insulin. This can cause blood glucose levels to

be high, and therefore, your insulin requirements can be high, too.

There are many ways of coping with stress. For example, people eat too much, sleep too much, or drink too much to cope with stress, but those are attempts to escape, not to cope. They cause more problems for you. Learn some healthy coping skills, such as walking, yoga, deep breathing, or listening to music, and figure out how you want to deal with stressful times.

Where do you go from here?

By now you are comfortable with carb counting, but after all this practice, there will be times that you find your insulin:carb ratio is not quite right, and your blood sugar levels are higher than your target ranges. What can you do about it? Always start with the basics. Measure the serving size and the amount of carbohydrate in it. Check your weighing and measuring of foods and see if your portions have grown or shrunk. Review your label reading and inter-pretation skills and check those for accuracy. Are you get-ting more physically fit? Muscles burn sugar even at rest.

Look at your medications. Review your background or basal insulin dose with your diabetes care provider. If that dose is what it should be, then review your insulin:carb ratio as well. These quality assurance checks every so often are very helpful and give you the support you need to suc-ceed with your diabetes care. Balancing your food, medica-tion, and exercise to control your blood sugar is a daily challenge, but now you have a record of your many experi-ences to take the guesswork out of diabetes management. With carb counting, you can take better care of your dia-betes and yourself.

Insulin pens are easy to use. You dial the dose, insert the needle, push the button to inject insulin, and hold. Done! If you are on MDI, an insulin pen is a good option to consider. Insulin pens make it easier to inject anytime, anywhere in your busy day. People who take three or more shots per day like to use them for their convenience and flexibility, even if you only use them at lunchtime. They are the size of a large fountain pen. For reusable pens, you can buy insulin in cartridges instead of vials.

You may want to try a pen if you:

- vary how much insulin you take based on what you eat

- want and need the flexibility and convenience of carrying your insulin with you

- want a quick, easy, and accurate insulin dose

- don't mind taking extra shots (note: you can't mix 2 types of insulin in one pen)

- have problems drawing up a dose of insulin due to poor eyesight or shaky hands

Discuss switching to a pen with your health care provider. Learn proper use of the pen and pen needles and proper storage for them.

What do you need to know about needles, pen needles, and syringes?
When you buy insulin syringes or pen needles, you make decisions about the needle length, the needle

gauge, and the size of the syringe. You'll find that syringes and pen needles come in various lengths and gauges. Common syringe sizes are 30 gauge with a short needle and 29 gauge with a standard needle. Common pen needle sizes are 31 gauge with a short needle and 29 gauge with a standard needle.

Needle gauge. Needles are made in four common gauges: 28, 29, 30, and 31. That's the diameter (width) of the needle. The higher the number the thinner the needle. Different companies make needles in different gauges. The thinnest needle on an insulin syringe is 30 gauge; the thinnest pen needle is 31 gauge.

Syringe size. There are three sizes of insulin syringe: 3/10 cc (holds 30 units), 1/2 cc (holds 50 units), and 1 cc (holds 100 units).

If you take:

• less than 30 units total at one time, use a 3/10 cc syringe

• between 30 and 50 units total at one time, use a 1/2 cc syringe

• between 50 and 100 units total at one time, use a 1 cc syringe

(Note: on the 3/10 and 1/2 cc syringes, each line equals one unit of insulin. On the 1 cc syringe, each line equals two units.)

13

Cornerstones
Knowledge and Support

Each person builds good control of their diabetes one experience at a time. But you can't build it by yourself. The cornerstones you build on are so important; it's difficult to understand why we don't pay enough attention to them. To succeed at taking care of your diabetes you need knowledge and support—knowledge to take care of your diabetes day to day and support to keep on keepin' on, even when your motivation is burnt out. Knowledgeable health care professionals can offer knowledge and serve as your coaches and offer support in their role as your cheerleaders. Your family members and friends can also support you and celebrate your progress in meeting the challenges before you. Look for help and you will find coaches and cheerleaders to offer you knowledge and support throughout the years and efforts to manage your diabetes.

Find Your Carb Counting Coach

If you decide carb counting is for you, you can begin a hunt for a carb counting coach by looking for a registered dietitian (RD) who is also a certified diabetes educator (CDE). This isn't a must, but a RD, CDE, should be able to help you master basic and advanced carbohydrate counting. How do you find a RD, CDE? This depends on where you live and how electronically connected you are. Try one or all of the following phone numbers or websites.

- **American Diabetes Association (ADA) Recognized Diabetes Education Programs.** ADA has a process for certifying diabetes education programs across the country. Going to one of these programs assures that you receive quality diabetes education and also assures that an RD is employed by the program. It is likely that the RD is also a CDE. These programs usually offer diabetes education group classes and one-to-one counseling. The people who provide the education are usually nurses and dietitians. Some programs may also have exercise physiologists, pharmacists, or behavioral counselors. There are nearly 1,900 ADA Recognized Diabetes Education programs in the country.

  Here are two ways to find programs in your area: Call the ADA at 1-800-DIABETES (1-800-342-2383). Ask for the program nearest you. On the Internet, look at the ADA website at www.diabetes.org and go to the list of recognized programs in your area. Or you can go directly to recognized programs at www.diabetes.org/education/eduprogram.asp.

- **American Association of Diabetes Educators (AADE)** provides you with two routes to find a diabetes educator—about a third are RDs. AADE is an association of nearly 11,000 health professionals who provide diabetes education. Diabetes educators may be nurses, nurse practitioners, dietitians, exercise physiologists, pharmacists, social workers, behavioral counselors, or psychologists. Diabetes educators are typically found at hospitals providing their services both in the hospital and to outpatients, at managed care organizations, in endocrinologists' offices, in large group-physician practices, at their own independent facilities, and more. Many diabetes educators choose to become a Certified Diabetes Educator (CDE). They take a certification exam every 5 years after they have a certain number of hours working with people with diabetes.

Here are two ways to find a diabetes educator. Call AADE at 1-800-TEAMUP4 (1-800-832-6874). The person who answers the phone will ask for your zip code and then will give you the names of some diabetes educators in your area. On the Internet, go to the AADE home page at www.diabeteseducators.org or www.aadenet.org and look for the "Find a Diabetes Educator" page. Click on the state in which you want to find an educator. Then a list of the diabetes educators in your state will come up.

■ **Yellow Pages.** You might find diabetes programs or registered dietitians at your local hospital or listed in the yellow pages. Look up "Endocrinologist" under "Physicians" in the Yellow Pages. Call and ask if they know of diabetes education programs or diabetes educators who are dietitians in your area.

■ **Talk to people.** Talk to people who have diabetes or people in your support group to see if they can recommend a health professional.

Do you know the questions to ask?

Once you have the names of a couple of diabetes educators, call and ask them a few questions about carbohydrate counting. You want to make sure you get what you are looking for. Tell them you want to learn either basic or advanced carbohydrate counting and why.

■ Ask if they teach carbohydrate counting and what types.

■ Ask about their breadth of experience.

- Ask how many sessions they think it will take for you to master carb counting.

- Ask about the cost of a session or the program.

- Ask whether they bill your health plan or must you submit the claim to your health care plan?

Is diabetes nutrition counseling covered by health insurance?

For starters, there's no single answer to the question "Does your health plan cover diabetes education, including nutrition counseling?" The answer depends on your health coverage and the regulations—either state or Federal—that apply to your health coverage. Traditionally, nutrition counseling, also referred to as *medical nutrition therapy*, has not been covered by health insurance plans. However, the frequency and amount of coverage for diabetes nutrition counseling, which includes carbohydrate counting, continues to change for the better. This means that more health plans are getting smart and saying yes to coverage of nutrition counseling.

To date, 42 states have passed legislation mandating that private insurance policies and managed care plans, which must follow that state's laws, cover medical nutrition therapy for state residents with diabetes. Call ADA to see if your state has a law or go on the Internet and click on your state. While the content of the laws varies widely, most laws cover people with type 1, type 2, or gestational diabetes. Most of the laws specifically mention "medical nutrition therapy" as a covered service. You should know, however, that these laws only cover about 30% of the population. The rest of the population is covered by Medicare or employer health plans, about 10% by Medicaid, or they don't have health insurance.

There are some loopholes to these state laws. If your insurance is through an employer and the health plan is "self-insured," then the health plan doesn't have to follow the state law noted above.

If you have Medicare part B (services provided outside of the hospital), you should be able to get your nutrition counseling covered if you get it at a diabetes program that can bill Medicare for diabetes education (mainly ADA Recognized education programs). Contact your local Medicare office by phone or go to www.Medicare.gov to find diabetes education programs that can bill Medicare.

If you are on Medicaid, the answer will differ from state to state. Medicaid is both a Federal and a state program. It is best that you ask what diabetes nutrition counseling will be covered.

If you are covered by the Federal Employee Health Benefits Plan (FEHBP), the answer is different depending on which plan you have. Again ask your health benefits manager if your plan covers diabetes nutrition counseling and if so, how much. FEHBP has recently improved their coverage of diabetes education.

Most HMOs and PPO plans require you to have your physician refer you to a dietitian, and you need pre-authorization before you go. Many have on-site RDs and diabetes education programs.

The bottom line: find out if your health plan covers diabetes nutrition counseling. If you feel you should be covered for diabetes education but your health plan is denying you this coverage, then ask questions and demand answers. Plead your case with the appropriate people. And gather other people with diabetes so you are many voices, not just one.

If you do not have a health plan that covers nutrition counseling or you have no health insurance at all, then the choice is yours as to whether to reach into your pocket and pay for nutrition counseling. It will be money well spent—and not that expensive when compared to medications, hospitalizations, or even the cost of a restaurant meal. The cost of a nutrition counseling session varies widely from about

$50 to $150. Some dietitians offer a package that includes a number of classes for one price.

Forming Your Cheerleading Squad

Beyond the how-to skills and knowledge, you need support when it comes to managing the day-to-day challenges of taking care of diabetes. There will be times that you are gung-ho and feel your carb counting efforts are paying off and other times where you just don't see the point in trying to control your blood glucose because nothing you do seems to work. Yes, you need diabetes educators to help you learn and to answer your questions, but you also need them to be part of your cheerleading squad. You need to be able to reach out to them when you need a shoulder to cry on, to brainstorm ideas for working out challenges, to solve day-to-day management problems, or to get a pat on the back when you hit your target goals.

Continue to see your educator after you complete your initial training. Perhaps you come in once or twice a year with a list of questions because you want more information about a particular topic, or your life situation has changed (pregnancy, going to college, retirement, etc.), or you are concerned that your diabetes is not as much in control as you want it to be. Another way to stay connected with your diabetes educators is to attend a diabetes support group or an insulin pump support group offered by your diabetes educators. In this environment, you not only get support from your educators, but you also encounter cheerleaders in the other members of the group as well. And you get to be a cheerleader too.

How do you keep on keepin' on?

One of the most difficult parts of diabetes is staying motivated to keep doing the daily tasks to take good care of yourself—counting carbohydrates, checking blood glucose several times a day, making medication decisions, taking the medications, checking your feet, and on and on. It is easy to suffer from "diabetes burnout." In his book *Diabetes Burnout* (ADA, 1999), William Polonsky, PhD, CDE, emphasizes the importance of getting educated and to keep being educated about diabetes. He states, "Acquiring knowledge and problem-solving skills can provide you with the hope and confidence that is needed to become a good problem-focused cope-er. Because diabetes knowledge is constantly expanding, it is important to stay informed as well. Diabetes support groups and relevant magazines (such as ADA's *Diabetes Forecast*) are likely to be good resources for you."

So, find your coaches (diabetes educators and physicians) and use them as you continue to learn and brainstorm to solve problems or deal with unusual situations. Let these health professionals become members of your cheerleading squad. Also reach out to other people with diabetes. You can find them through a local diabetes support group or try searching diabetes-related Internet sites that may offer chat rooms that appeal to you.

Dr. Polonsky ends *Diabetes Burnout* with a quote that we think is also an appropriate end to this book. "The fundamental lesson to remember is that feeling stressed about living with diabetes is normal, feeling at war with diabetes is common, but problematic feelings like these can be conquered. With attention, kindness, and humor, you can overcome diabetes burnout and make peace with diabetes. This is not to suggest that you and diabetes will ever become the best of friends, but you can learn to make room for diabetes in your life. And, as you are certain to discover, this will actually improve the quality, and perhaps even quantity, of your life."

Meet Maddie

Maddie is a 71-year-old retired elementary school math teacher. She has had type 2 diabetes for about 16 years. She has taken moderately good care of her diabetes. Her HbA_{1c}

levels have been between 8–9% over the years, but the last two have been closer to 9%. Unfortunately, she just discovered that her blood pressure is high enough that she needs a blood pressure medication. In addition, she found out she is spilling a small amount of protein in her urine. Maddie is concerned, frustrated, and feeling down about her diabetes. She feels she does a lot to manage her diabetes day to day, but she continues to have a number of high blood glucose levels each week. When Maddie was first diagnosed with diabetes, she received some education from her doctor and a dietitian. During a few sessions, the dietitian taught Maddie how to use basic carb counting. Maddie was comfortable with this, however she was growing tired of the similarity of her meals and the lack of flexibility in her meal plan. For many years Maddie has been taking two types of diabetes pills. She has progressively taken larger doses and is now taking the maximum dose of each. Maddie's doctor has been telling her that she really needs to think about starting insulin to control her blood glucose levels. Maddie has put her doctor off several times by bargaining for more time to "do better on her meal plan." One day Maddie was reading the health section in the local paper. She saw the announcement of a diabetes support group for people with diabetes who take insulin. Maddie decided to attend the next group. She figured that she might get the true lowdown on insulin from people who take it.

When Maddie introduced herself to the group, she let people know she didn't yet take insulin, but her doctor was recommending that she do so. When the group ended, a women came over to talk with her. She said that she had been in a similar situation about 6 months ago, but she finally bit the bullet and went on insulin. She said she had been amazed at how easy it is to give herself insulin, how much better she now feels, and how much more in control her blood glucose levels are. The woman noted her HbA_{1c} has gone from 9.3 to 8.2% in 6 months. This woman also suggested Maddie go see the dietitian at the local hospital diabetes education program. The woman told Maddie that in three sessions, they taught her to do advanced carb counting. She said now she is able to adjust her insulin dose based on her blood glucose levels and what she plans to eat. The woman noted that she ended up paying for the sessions herself because her health plan would not, but she added it was not that expensive and was well worth it. Maddie felt she had found a new friend—someone who understood her situation. That made her feel good. She vowed to come back to the group's next meeting. She also promised herself she would wake up the next morning and call her doctor to let her know she was ready to go on insulin and call the RD to schedule an appointment. Maddie was feeling a bit more positive about her ability and options to get her blood glucose under control.

Carb Counts of Everyday Foods

Starches

(includes breads, cereals, grains, starchy vegetables, crackers, snacks, beans, peas, lentils, and starchy foods prepared with fat)
The average grams of carbohydrate per serving = 15 g
The average calories per serving = 80 (this is not true for foods prepared with fat).

Starches	Serving	Calories	Carb (g)	Fiber (g)
Breads				
Bagel	1/2 (35 g)	98	19	1
Bread, pumpernickel	1 slice	80	15	2
Bread, rye	1 slice	83	16	2
Bread, white, reduced-calorie	2 slices	96	20	4
Bread, white, French, Italian	1 slice	67	12	1
Bread, whole-wheat	1 slice	70	13	2
Bread sticks	2	82	14	1
English muffin	1/2	67	13	1
Hamburger bun	1/2	61	11	1
Hot dog bun	1/2	61	11	1
Pita bread (6" dia.)	1/2	83	17	1
Raisin bread	1 slice	71	14	1

Starches	Serving	Calories	Carb (g)	Fiber (g)
Roll, plain	1	85	14	1
Tortilla, corn, 6–7"	1	56	12	1
Tortilla, flour, 7–8"	1	114	20	1
Waffle, reduced-fat, 4 1/2" square	1	80	16	1
Cereals, cold				
All Bran	1/2 cup	75	22	10
Bran Buds	1/2 cup	112	33	16
Cheerios	3/4 cup	90	16	2
Cornflakes	3/4 cup	89	20	1
Granola, low-fat	1/2 cup	105	21	2
Grape nuts	1/4 cup	105	24	2
Grapenut flakes	3/4 cup	104	24	3
Kix	3/4 cup	66	14	0
Product 19	3/4 cup	88	20	1
Puffed rice	1 1/2 cup	90	22	0
Puffed Wheat	1 1/2 cup	76	15	1
Raisin bran	1/2 cup	85	22	4
Rice Krispies	3/4 cup	71	16	0
Shredded Wheat	1/2 cup	90	20	2
Sugar frosted flakes	1/2 cup	67	16	0
Wheaties	3/4 cup	80	18	2
Cereals, cooked				
Cream of rice	1/2 cup	63	14	0
Cream of wheat	1/2 cup	67	14	1
Grits	1/2 cup	73	16	0
Oatmeal	1/2 cup	73	13	2
Whole wheat	1/2 cup	75	17	2

Starches	Serving	Calories	Carb (g)	Fiber (g)
Crackers and Snacks				
Animal crackers	8	89	15	0
Crispbread	2 slices	73	16	3
Graham crackers	3	89	16	1
Matzos	3/4 oz	83	18	1
Melba toast	4 slices	78	15	1
Oyster crackers	24	78	13	0
Popcorn, popped, no fat added	3 cups	92	19	4
Popcorn, microwave, light	3 cups (1/2 bag)	65	11	2
Pretzels, sticks/rings	3/4 oz	80	17	1
Rice cake, regular	2	70	15	1
Rye crisp	3 slices	86	20	2
Tortilla chips, not fried	17	82	18	3
Triscuits, reduced fat	5 wafers	81	15	2
Grains				
Bulgur, cooked	1/2 cup	76	17	4
Cornmeal, dry, degermed	3 Tbsp	97	20	2
Couscous, cooked	1/3 cup	67	14	1
Flour, white	3 Tbsp	87	18	1
Kasha	1/2 cup	91	20	2
Millet, cooked	1/4 cup	72	14	1
Rice, white, long grain, cooked	1/3 cup	69	15	0
Rice, brown, cooked	1/3 cup	72	15	1
Wheat germ, toasted	3 Tbsp	80	10	3

Starches	Serving	Calories	Carb (g)	Fiber (g)
Pasta				
Macaroni, cooked firm	1/2 cup	99	20	1
Noodles, enriched egg, cooked	1/2 cup	106	20	1
Spaghetti, cooked firm	1/2 cup	99	20	1
Dried Beans, Peas, Lentils				
Beans				
Baked	1/3 cup	79	17	4
Garbanzo (chickpeas), cooked	1/2 cup	134	22	4
Kidney, canned	1/2 cup	105	19	4
Kidney, cooked	1/2 cup	112	20	6
Lima	2/3 cup	114	21	8
Lima, canned	2/3 cup	125	23	5
Navy, cooked	1/2 cup	129	24	6
Pinto, cooked	1/2 cup	117	22	7
White, cooked	1/2 cup	126	23	6
Lentils, cooked	1/2 cup	117	20	8
Miso (sodium)	3 Tbsp	106	14	3
Peas, split, cooked	1/2 cup	117	21	8
Peas, black-eyed, cooked	1/2 cup	100	18	6
Starchy Vegetables				
Corn, frozen, cooked	1/2 cup	66	17	2
Corn, whole kernel, vac. pack	1/2 cup	83	20	2
Corn on cob, cooked, medium	1 cob (5 oz)	83	19	2
Corn on cob, frozen, 3"	1 cob	70	14	1
Mixed vegetables with corn	1 cup	80	18	4

Starches	Serving	Calories	Carb (g)	Fiber (g)
Mixed vegetables with pasta	1 cup	80	15	5
Peas, green, canned, drained	1/2 cup	59	11	4
Peas, green, frozen, cooked	1/2 cup	62	11	4
Plantain, cooked slices	1/2 cup	89	24	2
Potato, baked with skin	3 oz	93	22	2
Potato, white, peeled, boiled	3 oz	73	17	2
Potato, mashed, flakes (with milk and fat)	1/2 cup	119	16	2
Squash, winter	1 cup	83	22	7
Potato, sweet, canned, vac. pack, pieces	1/2 cup	92	22	3
Yam, plain	1/2 cup	79	19	2

(sodium) = 400 mg or more of sodium per exchange.

Vegetables

(includes raw, fresh, and canned vegetables and vegetable juices)
The average grams of carbohydrate per serving = 5 g

Vegetables	Serving	Calories	Carb (g)	Fiber (g)
Artichoke, cooked	1/2	30	7	3
Artichoke hearts	1/2 cup	36	7	0
Asparagus, frozen	1/2 cup	23	4	3
Asparagus spears, canned, drained	1/2 cup	23	3	2
Beans (green, wax), canned, drained	1/2 cup	14	3	1
Beans, snap, frozen	1/2 cup	18	4	2
Bean sprouts, raw	1 cup	31	6	2
Beets, canned, sliced, drained	1/2 cup	26	6	2
Broccoli, raw, chopped	1 cup	25	5	3
Broccoli spears, frozen	1/2 cup	26	5	3
Brussels sprouts, frozen, cooked	1/2 cup	33	6	3
Cabbage, cooked	1/2 cup	16	3	2
Cabbage, Chinese, raw	1 cup	12	2	1
Cabbage, green, raw	1 cup	18	4	2
Carrots, canned, drained	1/2 cup	17	4	1
Carrots, cooked	1/2 cup	35	8	3
Carrots, raw	1 cup	47	11	3
Cauliflower, frozen, cooked	1/2 cup	17	3	2
Cauliflower, raw	1 cup	25	5	2
Celery, cooked	1/2 cup	14	3	1
Celery, raw	1 cup	19	4	2

Vegetables	Serving	Calories	Carb (g)	Fiber (g)
Cucumber, raw	1 cup	14	3	1
Eggplant, cooked	1/2 cup	13	3	1
Endive/escarole, raw	1 cup	9	2	2
Greens, cooked				
Collard	1/2 cup	17	4	1
Kale	1/2 cup	21	4	1
Mustard	1/2 cup	10	2	1
Turnip	1/2 cup	14	3	2
Kohlrabi, cooked	1/2 cup	24	6	1
Lettuce, iceberg	1 cup	7	1	1
Mixed vegetables (no corn, peas, pasta)	1/2 cup	20	3	1
Mushrooms, canned, drained	1/2 cup	19	4	2
Mushrooms, fresh, cooked	1/2 cup	21	4	2
Mushrooms, raw	1 cup	18	3	1
Okra, frozen, cooked	1/2 cup	34	8	3
Onions, chopped, cooked	1/2 cup	46	11	2
Onions, raw	1 cup	61	14	3
Onion, green, raw	1 cup	32	7	3
Pea pods, cooked	1/2 cup	34	6	2
Pea pods, raw	1 cup	61	11	4
Pepper, green, cooked	1/2 cup	19	5	1
Pepper, green, raw	1 cup	27	6	2
Pepper, hot green chile, raw	1 cup	60	14	2
Radishes	1 cup	20	4	2
Romaine	1 cup	9	1	1

Vegetables	Serving	Calories	Carb (g)	Fiber (g)
Sauerkraut, canned (sodium)	1/2 cup	22	5	3
Spinach, canned, drained	1/2 cup	25	4	3
Spinach, frozen, cooked	1/2 cup	27	5	3
Spinach, raw	1 cup	12	2	2
Squash, summer, cooked	1/2 cup	18	4	1
Squash, summer, raw	1 cup	26	6	2
Tomatoes, canned, solids and liquids	1/2 cup	24	5	1
Tomatoes, raw	1 cup	38	8	2
Tomato juice (sodium)	1/2 cup	21	5	0
Tomato sauce (sodium)	1/2 cup	37	9	2
Turnips, cooked, cubed	1/2 cup	14	4	2
Vegetable juice (sodium)	1/2 cup	23	6	1
Water chestnuts	1/2 cup	35	9	2
Watercress, raw	1 cup	4	0	0
Zucchini, raw	1 cup	18	4	2
Zucchini squash, sliced, cooked	1/2 cup	14	4	1

(sodium) = 400 mg or more of sodium per exchange.

Fruit

(includes fresh, dried, canned, and frozen fruit; and fruit juices)
The average grams of carbohydrate per serving = 15 g

Fruit	Serving	Calories	Carb (g)	Fiber (g)
Fruit, fresh				
Apple, unpeeled, small	1 (4 oz)	63	16	3
Apricots	4	68	16	3
Banana, small	1 (4 oz)	64	16	2
Blackberries	3/4 cup	56	14	5
Blueberries	3/4 cup	61	15	3
Cantaloupe	1 cup	56	13	1
Cherries, sweet	12 (3 oz)	59	14	2
Cranberries	1 cup	47	12	4
Figs, large	1 1/2	71	18	3
Grapefruit	1/2	51	13	2
Grapes, seedless	17	60	15	1
Honeydew melon	1 cup	59	16	1
Kiwi	1	56	14	3
Mango	1/2 cup	68	18	2
Nectarine	1	67	16	2
Orange	1 (6 1/2 oz)	62	15	3
Papaya	1 cup	55	14	3
Peach, medium	1 (6 oz)	57	15	3
Pear, large	1/2 (4 oz)	59	15	2
Pineapple	3/4 cup	57	14	1
Plums, small	2 (5 oz)	73	17	2
Raspberries, black, red	1 cup	60	14	8
Rhubarb	2 cups	52	11	4
Strawberries	1 1/4 cups	56	13	4

Fruit	Serving	Calories	Carb (g)	Fiber (g)
Tangerine, small	2 (8 oz)	74	19	3
Watermelon, cubed	1 1/4 cups	64	14	1
Fruit, canned or jarred, with some juice				
Applesauce, unsweetened	1/2 cup	52	14	2
Apricots	1/2 cup	60	15	2
Cherries, sweet, juice packed	1/2 cup	68	17	1
Cranberry sauce	1/4 cup	86	22	1
Fruit cocktail, juice packed	1/2 cup	57	15	1
Fruit cocktail	1/2 cup	55	14	1
Grapefruit, juice packed	3/4 cup	69	17	1
Mandarin oranges	3/4 cup	69	18	1
Peaches, juice packed	1/2 cup	55	14	1
Pears, juice packed	1/2 cup	62	16	3
Pineapple, juice packed	1/2 cup	74	20	1
Plums, juice packed	1/2 cup	73	19	1
Pumpkin, solid packed	3/4 cup	59	15	6
Fruit, dried				
Apples, rings	4	63	17	2
Apricots, halves	8	66	17	3
Dates	3	68	18	2
Figs	1 1/2	71	18	3
Fruit snacks, chewy, roll	1	78	18	1
Prunes, uncooked	3	60	16	2
Raisins, dark, seedless	2 Tbsp	54	14	1

Fruit	Serving	Calories	Carb (g)	Fiber (g)
Fruit, frozen unsweetened				
Blackberries	3/4 cup	73	18	6
Blueberries	3/4 cup	58	14	3
Melon balls	1 cup	57	14	1
Raspberries	1/2 cup	61	15	6
Strawberries	1 1/4 cups	65	17	4
Fruit juices				
Apple juice/cider	1/2 cup	58	15	0
Apricot nectar	1/2 cup	70	17	0
Cranapple juice cocktail	1/3 cup	53	13	0
Cranberry juice cocktail	1/3 cup	48	12	0
Fruit juice bars, 100% juice	1	75	19	0
Grape juice	1/3 cup	51	13	0
Orange juice, fresh	1/2 cup	56	13	0
Orange juice, from frozen	1/2 cup	56	13	0
Pineapple juice, canned	1/2 cup	70	17	0
Prune juice	1/3 cup	60	15	1

Sweets and Sugary Foods

The grams of carbohydrate per serving in this group vary quite a bit. The fat and calorie content vary quite a bit too.

Sweets	Serving	Calories	Carb (g)	Fat (g)
Angel food cake	1/12 cake	142	32	0
Brownie, unfrosted	2" sq	115	18	4.5
Cake, unfrosted	2" sq	97	17	3
Cake, frosted	2" sq	175	29	6.5
Cupcake, frosted, small	1	172	28	6
Donut, plain cake	1	198	23	11
Donut, glazed (3 3/4" dia.)	2 oz	245	27	14
Fruit spreads, 100% fruit	1 Tbsp	43	11	0
Gelatin, reg. (Jello)	1/2 cup	80	19	0
Gingersnaps	3	87	16	2
Granola bar	1	133	18	5.5
Granola bar, fat-free	1	140	35	0
Honey	1 Tbsp	64	17	0
Ice cream, light	1/2 cup	100	14	4
Ice cream, fat-free, no sugar added	1/2 cup	90	20	0
Jam or preserves, regular	1 Tbsp	48	13	0
Jelly, regular	1 Tbsp	52	14	0
Pie, fruit, 2 crusts	1/6 pie	290	43	13
Pie, pumpkin or custard	1/8 pie	168	19	8.5
Pudding, regular, low-fat milk	1/2 cup	144	26	2.5

Sweets	Serving	Calories	Carb (g)	Fiber (g)
Pudding, sugar-free, low-fat milk	1/2 cup	90	13	2
Sherbet	1/2 cup	132	29	2
Sorbet	1/2 cup	130	31	0
Sweet roll or Danish	1 (2 1/2 oz)	263	36	11
Syrup, maple, regular	1 Tbsp	52	13	0
Syrup, pancake, light	2 Tbsp	49	13	0
Syrup, pancake, regular	1 Tbsp	57	15	0
Vanilla wafers	5	88	15	3
Yogurt, frozen, fat-free	1/3 cup	60	12	0
Yogurt, frozen, fat-free, no sugar added	1/2 cup	90	18	0

Milk and Yogurt

The average grams of carbohydrate per serving = 12 g

Milks and milk products	Serving	Calories	Carb (g)	Total fat (g)
Nonfat or Very Low-fat				
Buttermilk, low-fat/fat-free	1 cup	99	12	2
Evaporated fat-free milk	1/2 cup	100	14	0.5
Milk, dry, fat-free	1/3 cup	82	12	0
Milk, fat-free	1 cup	86	12	0.5
Milk, 1%	1 cup	102	12	2.5
Yogurt, nonfat, plain	3/4 cup (6 oz)	90	13	0
Yogurt, nonfat, fruit-flavored, nonnutritive sweetener	1 cup	100	17	0
Low-fat				
Milk, 2%	1 cup	121	12	4.5
Sweet acidophilus milk	1 cup	110	12	3.5
Yogurt, low-fat, plain	3/4 cup (6 oz)	112	13	3
Yogurt, low-fat, with fruit	1 cup	253	47	3
Whole				
Whole milk	1 cup	150	11	8
Evaporated milk	1/2 cup	169	13	10
Goat's milk, whole	1 cup	168	11	10

Meat and Other Foods that Contain Mainly Protein and Fat

Most of the foods in this group—meats, poultry, seafood, eggs—contain no carbohydrate. However, several foods in this food group—processed meats, tofu, cheeses, and peanut butter—contain very small amounts of carbohydrate.

	Serving	Calories	Carb (g)	Total fat (g)
Meat				
Beef, jerky, dried (sodium)	1 oz	94	4	4
Fish sticks (2)		152	13	7
Meat sticks, smoked	1 oz	153	15	14
Tempeh	1/4 cup	83	7	3
Tofu	1/2 cup	94	2	6
Cheese				
Cheese, fat-free	1 oz	37	3	0
Cottage cheese, nonfat	1/4 cup	35	3	0
Ricotta, part-skim	1/4 cup	86	3	5
Processed American cheese, fat-free	3/4 oz slice	30	2	0
Peanut butter, chunky	1 Tbsp	94	4	8
Peanut butter, smooth	1 Tbsp	94	3	8

Fats

Many of the foods in this group—margarine, butter, oils, olives, bacon, and sausage—contain no carbohydrate. Several foods in this food group—nuts, salad dressings, low-fat and fat-free mayonnaise, and spreads—contain very small amounts of carbohydrate.

	Serving	Calories	Carb (g)	Total fat (g)
Nuts				
Almonds	1 oz	165	6	15
Cashews	1 oz	161	9	13
Peanuts	1 oz	165	5	14
Pecans	1 oz	189	5	19
Pumpkin seeds	1 oz	126	15	6
Walnuts	1 oz	182	5	18
Salad Dressings				
Salad dressing, fat-free	1 Tbsp	20	5	0
Salad dressing, reduced-fat	2 Tbsp	80	5	6
Salad dressing, regular	1 Tbsp	64	2	6
Mayonnaise				
Mayonnaise, fat-free	1 Tbsp	10	2	0
Mayonnaise, reduced-fat	1 Tbsp	40	3	3

Alcohol

Note: Most of the calories in alcoholic beverages are provided by the alcohol. Most alcoholic beverages contain no carbohydrate, but other beverages do. When you drink alcohol, be careful because alcohol can either make your blood glucose rise or fall too low. See page 155 about the use of alcoholic beverages.

Beverage	Serving	Carbohydrate (grams)
Beer (regular)	12 oz	13*
Beer (light)	12 oz	5*
Brandy	1 1/2 oz (1 shot)	0
Liquor (any type; for example, gin, rum, vodka)	1 1/2 oz (1 shot)	0
Liqueur (any type, for example, Kahlua, creme de menthe)	1 1/2 oz (1 shot)	14–18*
Wine (white)	4 oz	1*
Wine (red)	4 oz	3*

* These are average numbers. Check the carbohydrate count for the specific alcoholic beverage you choose from a nutrient database. Nutrition Facts labels do not appear on alcoholic beverages.

Books and Resources

A lot of information is at your fingertips from food Nutrition Facts labels (chapter 8), but that information will not meet all your needs, especially when it comes to fresh produce, meats, prepared foods from the supermarket, and restaurant foods. The following resources will put more carb counts at your fingertips:

- Appendix 1—*The Carbohydrate Count of Everyday Foods*. On pages 172–188 there is a list of the carbohydrate content of 195 basic foods, from fresh and canned fruit to cereal and low-fat mayonnaise.

Books

- *The Diabetes Carbohydrate and Fat Gram Guide*, 2nd edition by LeaAnn Holzmeister, RD, CDE, American Diabetes Association, 2000.
  This book provides the carbohydrate count, as well as other nutrition information for thousands of foods, including fruits, vegetables, and other produce; meats, poultry, and seafood; desserts; many foods you know by their brand name; frozen entrées; and more.

- *The ADA Complete Guide to Convenience Food Counts* by LeaAnn Holzmeister, RD, CDE, American Diabetes Association, 2001.
This book provides the carbohydrate count, as well as other nutrition information for more than 4,000 foods including many grocery and deli prepared and convenience foods you know by their brand name; frozen entrées; and more.

- *The Complete Book of Food Counts,* 5th edition by Corinne T. Netzer, Dell Publishing, 2000.
This book provides the carbohydrate count, as well as other nutrition information for thousands of foods including fruits, vegetables, and other produce; meats, poultry, and seafood; desserts; many foods you know by their brand name; frozen entrees, and more.

- *The Corinne T. Netzer Carbohydrate Counter,* 2nd edition by Corinne T. Netzer, Dell Publishing, 1998.
This book provides the carbohydrate count, for thousands of foods including fruits, vegetables, and other produce; meats, poultry, and seafood; desserts; many foods you know by their brand name; frozen entrees, and more.

- *Calories and Carbohydrates,* 13th edition by Barbara Kraus, Mass Market Paperback, 1999.
This book provides the carbohydrate and calorie count for more than 8,000 foods including fruits, vegetables, and other produce; meats, poultry, and seafood; desserts; many foods you know by their brand name; frozen entrees, and more.

- *Bowes and Church Food Values of Portions Commonly Used,* 17th edition by Janet Pennington, J.P. Lippincott Company, 1998. To order call 1-800-777-2295. This book is a resource for complete nutrition information for most basic foods and many ingredients. It is 8 1/2" × 11", so it's not easy to carry with you.

■ *American Diabetes Association Guide to Healthy Restaurant Eating* by Hope Warshaw, MMSc, RD, CDE, American Diabetes Association, 1998. This guide provides the basics about diabetes nutrition management, meal planning goals, and strategies for healthy restaurant eating. There's nutrition information including carbohydrate, calories, fat, percent of calories as fat, saturated fat, cholesterol, sodium, fiber, and protein with servings or exchanges for more than 2,500 menu items from nearly 60 major restaurant chains. In addition, there are two healthy, well-balanced sample meals for each restaurant and checkmarks by the healthiest choices from each restaurant.

■ All cookbooks published by the American Diabetes Association. ADA publishes many diabetes cookbooks. The nutrition information for each recipe provides the grams of carbohydrate content per serving as well as fat, saturated fat, protein, cholesterol, sodium, and more.

Booklets

■ *Ethnic and Regional Food Practices Series.* The American Diabetes Association and The American Dietetic Association publish a series of 8 1/2" × 11" booklets designed to provide information about the habits, holidays, and foods of a wide variety of cultures. As someone who needs carbohydrate information for a wide variety of foods, you might find the carbohydrate information for ethnic foods in these booklets useful. The following titles are available: Indian and Pakistani, Cajun and Creole, Filipino American, Soul and Traditional Southern, Northern Plains Indian, Chinese American, Mexican American, Jewish, Alaskan Native, Navajo, and Hmong American.

Order from the American Dietetic Association at 1-800-366-1655.

Internet

- www.cyberdiet.com has a database of thousands foods with carbohydrate content as well as other nutrients. Basic foods, brand name, and restaurant foods are included.

- www.usda.gov/fnic/foodcomp is the site for the United States Department of Agriculture (USDA) nutrient database. (This nutrient database is the base of many commercial databases.) This database can be downloaded. A program allowing you to search the database is also available. The database is also available on CD-ROM and may be purchased from the Government Printing Office

Commercial Software

- Many commercial software programs are available that provide you with a nutrition database of commonly eaten foods. Make sure the one you purchase contains a sizable number of foods, at least 15,000, and includes the types of foods you eat.

Record Keeping Forms

Carbohydrate Counting and Blood Glucose Results Record

Day/Date: _____

Time/ meal	Diabetes medicines		Food		Carb count (choices/ grams)
	Type	Amount	Type	Amount	

Notes about day:

Blood glucose results

Fasting/ before b'fast/ time	After b'fast/ time	Before lunch/ time	After lunch/ time	Before dinner/ time	After dinner/ time	Before bed/ time	Other/ time

Sample

Carbohydrate Counting and Blood Glucose Results Record

Day/Date: _Tuesday, June 3_

Time/ meal	Diabetes medicines		Food		Carb count (choices/ grams)
	Type	Amount	Type	Amount	
6:45 a.m./ B'fast	N H	12 u 4 u	Shredded Wheat 'n Bran with Cheerios Milk Banana	1/2 cup 3/4 cup 1 cup 1 large	
12:30 p.m.	H	5 u	Sub sandwich– 12" turkey, ham, cheese, lettuce, tomato, onions, pickles, mustard Pretzels	1 2 1/2 oz bag	
5:00 p.m.			Apple	1 large	
7:15 p.m. Dinner	H	7 u			
10:00 p.m.	N	9 u			

Notes about day:
Went for a walk after dinner. Felt a bit low an hour after return (see other BG).

	Blood glucose results						
Fasting/ before b'fast/ time	After b'fast/ time	Before lunch/ time	After lunch/ time	Before dinner/ time	After dinner/ time	Before bed/ time	Other/ time
92/6:30	179/ 9:10						
		123/ 12:30	89/ 2:00				

Build Your Food and Carb Counting Database

As you begin to use carb counting to control your diabetes, you will find out the carb count of many foods—the crackers you buy, the apples you usually choose, your favorite ice cream, frozen entrée, recipe, or restaurant meal. Rather than having to keep a mental list of the carb counts of these foods or having to look them up every time, start to build your Carb Count Database. This information helps you keep track of the foods, the servings you usually eat, the carb count, and any notes you want to record. For example, maybe you find that a particular food does (or does not) make your blood glucose rise as much as you thought it would or a particular food is a good snack before exercise or on a full day of hiking.

You can keep this record in a notebook, a computer file, or on your handheld day timer. Keep it in a convenient place and in a format that works for you.

Carb Count Database

Food	Serving (amount I eat)	Carb choices/grams	Notes (effect on blood glucose level, what you would do next time you eat this, etc.)

Sample

Food	Serving (amount I eat)	Carb choices/grams	Notes
Bagel (Dunkin' Donuts)—pumpernickel	1	70	More carbs than I thought!
Grandma Grace's Apple Cobbler	3/4 cup	35 (from recipe analysis)	Don't need as much insulin as I thought I would to cover it.
Domino's cheese pizza with onions and mushrooms—hand tossed	2 14" pieces	45	Raises my blood glucose most 3 hours after I eat it.
Healthy Choice Ginger Chicken Hunan	1 entrée	59	Quick rise in blood glucose.
Weight Watcher's Garden Lasagna	1 entrée	30	Works well.

Here's another example of a chart you can use for your database of foods.

Food	My usual serving	Grams of carbohydrate	Notes about effect on BG level	Notes for next time I eat this food/meal

Sample

Food	My usual serving	Grams of carbohydrate	Notes about effect on BG level	Notes for next time I eat this food/meal
Dry Cereal Shredded Wheat 'n Bran mixed with Raisin Bran	1 cup (1/2 cup of each)	59	1 hour after eating— BG 185 2 hours after eating— BG 220	Decrease amount of cereal or take more rapid-acting insulin
McDonalds Quarter Pounder with small fries and 1% milk	1 1 1	37 26 13 —— 76	2 hours after eating— BG 165	Took 5 units of rapid-acting insulin to cover meal— worked well

Index

A

AADE. *See* American Association of Diabetes Educators

ACE inhibitors, 69

ADA. *See* American Diabetes Association

Advanced carb counting, 17, 20–21, 137–160

terminology of, 138–143

Alcohol

adjusting insulin for, 155

carb counts for, 186

Alpha-glucosidase inhibitors, 31

American Association of Diabetes Educators (AADE), 162–163

American Diabetes Association (ADA)

Recognized Diabetes Education programs, 162

recommendations from, 6, 10, 12–13, 69

Aspart, 32

B

Background insulin, 140–142

Basal insulin, 140–142

Basic carb counting, 17–20

Beans, carb counts for dried, 175

Biguanide, 52

Blood glucose levels

checking, 50, 54–55

correcting high, 148–149

correcting low, 151

factors affecting, 13–14, 55–56, 60, 63, 159–161

importance of controlling, 6–7, 26–27

postprandial, 143–145

predicting, 1–2

target ranges for, 7

variations in, 157–159

Blood glucose records

for finding insulin-to-carbohydrate ratio, 145–146, 152

the number 15 in, 21–22
resources for, 189–192
staying motivated,
  168–171
two methods of, 21
Crackers, carb counts for,
  174

D
D-phenylalanine, 31, 51
Daly, Anne, vii–viii
Dawn phenomenon, 140
DCCT. *See* Diabetes Control
  and Complications
  Trial
Diabetes, challenge of
  choosing food with, vii
Diabetes Burnout, 168–169
Diabetes Control and Com-
  plications Trial
  (DCCT), vii, 16
Diabetes educator
  locating, 163–165
  paying for, 166–167
  working with, 165–166
Diabetes medications,
  51–53
  adjusting, 20
  and hypoglycemia, 31
  keeping records of, 20
  recent developments in,
    30–32
Diabetes snack products,
  35–36
Diabetic kidney disease, 69
Diary. *See* Food diary;
  Record keeping

Dietary fiber, on food labels,
  90
Dietitian
  consulting with, 17–20,
    24, 72, 137–138
  getting coaching from,
    163–167
Dose, figuring for your
  insulin, 149–153

E
Eating habits. *See also*
  Record keeping
  observing, 39–46
Eating out, 100–113
Emotions. *See also* Stress
  effect on blood glucose
    levels, 56
Exchange System, 21

F
Fad diets, 15
Fast food, 107–108
Fat replacers, 74–75
Fats
  amount per serving, 4
  body's need for, 72
  carb counts for, 187
  counting, 60–68, 70–75
  different types of, 63,
    71–72
  effect on blood glucose
    levels, 63–67,
    155–156
  foods containing, 61–62
FDA. *See* Food and Drug
  Administration

counting, 60–70
effect on blood glucose
  levels, 63–67,
  155–156
and fad diets, 15
on food labels, 91
foods containing, 61–62
snacks containing, 35
Publications, for counting
  carbohydrates, 189–192

R
Rapid-acting insulin, 32, 53,
  141–142, 153–155
Raw meat, *versus* cooked,
  84, 103
RD. *See* Registered dietitian
  (RD)
RDAs. *See* Recommended
  Dietary Allowances
RDI. *See* Recommended
  Daily Intake levels
Recipes, combination,
  108–110
Recommended Daily Intake
  (RDI) levels, 91
Recommended Dietary
  Allowances (RDAs), 69
Record keeping, 5–6, 27–28,
  38–39, 47–50, 54–55
of blood glucose levels,
  47–50, 54–55,
  114–133
of diabetes medications,
  50
examples of, 118–131
forms for, 193–202

of restaurant meals,
  101–102
Reducing sugars, easy ways
  for, 11
Registered dietitian (RD),
  locating, 163–165
Repaglinide, 31–32, 51
Resources, for counting
  carbohydrates, 189–192
Restaurant meals, 100–113
keeping records of,
  101–102
tips for, 102–107, 113
Risk factors, 15, 69–72

S
Salad dressings, carb counts
  for, 187
Salt. *See* Sodium
Saturated fats, 63, 71
on food labels, 89
risks from, 15, 70–72
Sensitivity factor, insulin,
  using the rule of 1500,
  148–149
Serving size, 4–7, 22–25,
  76–86
on food labels, 89
measuring, 5, 28, 77–80
Servings per container, on
  food labels, 89
Short-acting insulin, 151
Snacks
and insulin use, 154–155
numbers of, 32–36
tips for, 34
Sodium, on food labels, 90

About the American Diabetes Association

The American Diabetes Association is the nation's leading voluntary health organization supporting diabetes research, information, and advocacy. Its mission is to prevent and cure diabetes and to improve the lives of all people affected by diabetes. The American Diabetes Association is the leading publisher of comprehensive diabetes information. Its huge library of practical and authoritative books for people with diabetes covers every aspect of self-care—cooking and nutrition, fitness, weight control, medications, complications, emotional issues, and general self-care.

To order American Diabetes Association books: Call 1-800-232-6733. http://store.diabetes.org [Note: there is no need to use **www** when typing this particular Web address]

To join the American Diabetes Association: Call 1-800-806-7801. www.diabetes.org/membership

For more information about diabetes or ADA programs and services: Call 1-800-342-2383. E-mail: Customerservice@diabetes.org www.diabetes.org

To locate an ADA/NCQA Recognized Provider of quality diabetes care in your area: Call 1-703-549-1500 ext. 2202. www.diabetes.org/recognition/Physicians/ListAll.asp

To find an ADA Recognized Education Program in your area: Call 1-888-232-0822. www.diabetes.org/recognition/education.asp

To join the fight to increase funding for diabetes research, end discrimination, and improve insurance coverage: Call 1-800-342-2383. www.diabetes.org/advocacy

To find out how you can get involved with the programs in your community: Call 1-800-342-2383. See below for program Web addresses.

- *American Diabetes Month:* Educational activities aimed at those diagnosed with diabetes—month of November. www.diabetes.org/ADM
- *American Diabetes Alert:* Annual public awareness campaign to find the undiagnosed—held the fourth Tuesday in March. www.diabetes.org/alert
- *The Diabetes Assistance & Resources Program (DAR):* diabetes awareness program targeted to the Latino community. www.diabetes.org/DAR
- *African American Program:* diabetes awareness program targeted to the African American community. www.diabetes.org/africanamerican
- *Awakening the Spirit: Pathways to Diabetes Prevention & Control:* diabetes awareness program targeted to the Native American community. www.diabetes.org/awakening

To find out about an important research project regarding type 2 diabetes: www.diabetes.org/ada/research.asp

To obtain information on making a planned gift or charitable bequest: Call 1-888-700-7029. www.diabetes.org/ada/plan.asp

To make a donation or memorial contribution: Call 1-800-342-2383. www.diabetes.org/ada/cont.asp